# BECOMING
# OPTIMAL
# YOU

## Dr. Dwight Bryan

becomingopt

First published 2022
ISBN: 978-1-7373684-0-3

Printed in the United States of America

*Dedication*

This book is dedicated to my family who have given me abundant love and support throughout the mountains and valleys of life. I am not nearly eloquent enough to express how much love and gratitude I feel for you. As is one of the major tenants of this book, I will spend every day of the rest of my life savoring the love and memories each of you have given me. You are always in my mind and in my heart.

I would like to also acknowledge the friends, neighbors, fellow students and co-workers who have nurtured me in so many ways for so many years. My memory bank is full of a vast array of conversations, events, good times as well as times of sorrow. I deeply treasure each of you — you've all impacted me in ways I can never describe.

Finally I'd like to mention and thank each and every patient who gave me the privilege to hear their story as their physician. They trusted me to do the best that I could to help them in their time of need. Each of those relationships were precious and I can never express how grateful I am for that honor.

I have been blessed in so many ways and I can only say thank you. I will spend every day trying to pay forward all the love and memories I have received.

With Deep Love and Gratitude,
Dwight

# INTRODUCTION

This book is the culmination of my personal journey to improve my health and wellness. Approximately 10–12 years ago, I began to realize that failure to correct my multiple personal health and well-being issues would not only shorten my life, but would add pain to those I had been trying to improve the lives of. Most, if not all of my issues, were a direct result of my lifestyle, a lack of personal attention to my own health, and my personal tendency to be a workaholic and overachiever. I was striving for my family to have what I perceived to be a better life than previous generations. I was oblivious to the price we were all paying.

By 2008, I had been a Board Certified Family Physician in practice for nearly 25 years. Most of this time I also had other outside business and professional activities. I'm sure my mother of southern roots would say I was burning the candle at both ends. The thumbnail story is I had run full speed for years, multitasking and overworking with little if any down time, family time, or me time. In addition, I ate the basic American diet of processed and fast foods, with little or no thought as to what nutrients my body required. I was so busy that I never really thought of—much less did— any exercise to speak of. At that point in my life I weighed very close to 350 pounds. I was a type 2 diabetic, very poorly controlled. I had a HbA1C of near 10.5 (with 5.7 or lower as normal) while I was taking medication for it. I had hypertension, multiple joint and back issues (with multiple surgeries, including a hip replacement), and high cholesterol.

The biggest issue happened as I was spending a month driving to and through the western United States on vacation with my wife. I developed massive bilateral pulmonary emboli. By the grace of God and the skills of two physicians in a 40-bed hospital in Bullhead City, Arizona, I survived.

While continuing to work and see patients, I began to realize that if something didn't change, the probability of my living to a ripe old age was very low. I decided to make a positive change in my life and health — for the benefit of my family as well as myself. During a family vacation one July, I told myself that when I got back home the change would begin the next month. I had continued to read, research, and digest all the information

I could to determine how to best improve my health and wellness. I was intrigued with what evidence-based techniques individuals could do in the vein of self-care to improve their health, wellness, and general satisfaction with their life. My studies included several medical educational programs focusing on health and wellness. The first one I attended was with The Cleveland Clinic Wellness Institute, directed at that time by the Chief Wellness Officer of The Cleveland Clinic, Mike Roizen, M.D. I also attended an educational program with The Benson-Henry Mind Body Medicine Institute, affiliated with Harvard Medical School. Finally, I attended a training and educational program with The Center for Mind Body Medicine of Washington, D.C. This Center is directed by Founder James Gordon, M.D. Dr. Gordon has served as Chairman of the White House committee on Integrative Medicine under both Presidents Bill Clinton and George W. Bush. The main work of this organization since its founding in 1991 has been to train individuals who then travel, when needed, to places all around the world to help individuals heal from catastrophe related trauma.

I continued to study many cutting-edge findings in the fields of nutrition, physical activity, and neurosciences — as well as general health and wellness. I began to apply what I was learning not only to my daily life as much as possible, but also to share the information with any individual or patient who I felt would benefit from it. I continued to research, write, and refine what worked for me as well as others.

There were significant challenges using this material in the setting of traditional healthcare. Although I did include it with patients as I could, today's practice of medicine is structured more toward procedures and medications— and the constant tapping of computer keys and getting the next patient through the door as quickly as possible. Money talks and you know what walks in the current American medical system. While I still love practicing medicine, this material is best suited to spending time and effort educating those you are helping. This requires spending enough time and developing a professional relationship and a genuine trust. This is best accomplished with a coaching or mentoring approach. What works is to help the client learn self-care techniques that will improve their lives in ways they cannot initially imagine.

As for me now, I feel more blessed every day than I deserve. My weight has stayed around the 200-pound mark for many years. All of my labs and vitals are excellent. My most recent Hemoglobin A1C level (6 months ago, as of this writing) was 4.9, and I've not taken diabetes medicine for years. My sense of joy in life and my appreciation of the many blessings I've known have never been better. I am much less stressed and impatient. I appreciate where I am, and I see the beauty around me at each and every moment. I am much better able to take the blows when life's challenges pop up, as they will for everyone. This program has helped me develop a resilience, allowing me to get up quicker each time life puts me down on the mat. It has changed me in ways I couldn't imagine in advance.

This book —and the organization I'm starting around it — is designed to help as many people as possible reach their full potential in life based on their desires and their willingness to do what it takes for them to get to where they would like to be. It's *your* life and *your* journey. No two journeys are identical. You live one day, one minute, and one second at a time. My greatest joy has been the honor and privilege to work with patients and other individuals to help them learn how to help themselves. This is my goal for whatever years left I may be blessed with on this earth. For each and every person who decides to make this effort, I'm very grateful. You will not only be helping yourself, but you may also witness an equally positive impact on those around you. My visualization of this is much like the pebble tossed into a pond and the circular ripple you see that moves out to all areas nearby.

## Scientific Evidence

There is a large body of scientific research that is fascinating and also validates what we will be working on in this 30-day workbook. Let me say from the start, we are presenting this workbook in such a way that even those with no interest in the underlying science can do very well with what they learn. I do think, though, it is important to lay out some of the very interesting and important scientific issues that we will be addressing with what you learn here. And of course for those who are interested, there are many available sources that present the actual research and data in much greater detail than is possible here.

## Chronic Inflammation

Inflammation forming in our body has a significant effect on our body's ability to fight off infections from bacteria, viruses, and other foreign invaders. It also plays a major role in our body's ability to mobilize healing from cuts, surgeries, or other physical insults. This activity is important in keeping us alive. We face a potentially large problem, however, when this system is hijacked by other issues occurring in the body — namely, *chronic inflammation*. When this occurs, and continues unabated, it significantly increases the risk of many serious diseases.

**What are some of these problems?**
1. Hypertension
2. Depression
3. Cardiovascular Disease
4. Cancers
5. Type 2 Diabetes
6. Asthma
7. Many Neurodegenerative Diseases, including Alzheimer's Disease
8. Can cause damage to your DNA

So, now that we have an idea what chronic inflammation is, as well as some of the serious problems it can lead to, let's consider the issues in our life that may be contributing to this often silent — but potentially deadly — problem.

**Some causes of chronic inflammation include:**
1. Smoking
2. Obesity
3. Chronic stress
4. Alcohol consumption
5. Lack of exercise
6. Eating processed foods

**Self-care techniques to decrease chronic inflammation include:**
1. Increase physical activity or movement
2. Practice stress reduction techniques
3. Anti-inflammatory diet
   - Increase plant consumption
   - Eat antioxidant rich foods
   - Consume foods rich in Omega 3 fatty acids
   - Eat less red meat and less processed foods

## Oxidative Damage in the Body

There is a natural chemical process in the body which causes the release of a particle known as a free radical. An excessive amount of these is problematic. As a real-world example, many of us have driven down the highway and have occasionally noticed large metal beams under an overpass with a significant amount of rusting. Sometimes we'll see road crews removing the rust and repairing the beams. This beam rusting is also oxidation, the same chemical reaction as what happens in your body. This is called *oxidative stress*. The oxidation in your body can cause significant damage over time, including damage to your DNA. This DNA damage will increase your rate of aging, as well as other medical and health issues.

**The question then becomes: How do you decrease this oxidative stress in your body?**

1. Avoid environmental pollutants
2. Eat a diet high in antioxidants, including an array of fruits and vegetables
3. Maintain your weight at your optimal level
4. Stay physically active with exercise and movement
5. Meditation correlates with lower oxidative stress

## DNA Telomeres

DNA is the molecule that contains our genetic code. This coding is passed from our parents to us at birth. This coding is very intricate and complex, and it is essential for all functions that occur in our body. At the end of each DNA molecule there is material called a *telomere*. A good analogy for you would be to visualize the plastic tips on the end of your shoelaces. Much like your shoelaces, with passage of time or other damage these telomeres shorten. This damage can be from things like the oxidative stress that we previously discussed. When shortening occurs it can lead to different diseases and ultimately death. So, as telomeres shorten, so does our life. The salient question here is what can we do to slow, stop, or even reverse this shortening?

As it turns out, many lifestyle choices have an impact on telomere length. Lifestyle behaviors that lead to shortening of your telomeres include:

1. Smoking
2. Obesity
3. Poor dietary choices

So, now we know some lifestyle choices that have a negative impact on both the quality of our life and the probable length of our life, based on our telomere length. Are there choices we can make that will maintain or even **lengthen your telomeres**? The short answer is, Yes. This list includes:

1. Consuming legumes, nuts, seaweed, fruits, coffee
2. Maintaining your optimal weight
3. Exercising
4. Decreasing your stress level
5. Meditating, which **lengthens your telomeres**

## Microbiome

Microbiome is more than a trillion bacteria that live mostly in our gastrointestinal tract, but also to a smaller degree on the skin and much less in other parts of the body. The gut microbiome has many benefits.

**What are some benefits of a balanced gut microbiome?**

1. It communicates with the brain on the production of neurotransmitters, such as serotonin and dopamine.
2. It helps in human development.
3. It plays a key role in the development of the immune system.
4. It helps in human nutrition, including the manufacture of several vitamins by the bacteria.

**How do we maximize the health of our microbiome?**

1. Eat plenty of vegetables and fruits.
2. Avoid processed foods and simple sugars as much as possible.
3. Consume sources of probiotics regularly.
4. Practice meditation — it significantly helps to regulate the bacteria in the gut, helps to suppress chronic inflammation, and regulates the stress response.
5. Avoid red meats.
6. Exercise regularly, which helps with maintaining a healthy microbiome by producing bacteria which make short chain fatty acids. These fatty acids have a host of health benefits.

## Neuroplasticity

At one time it was thought that by early in life the total number of brain cells and connections would have developed for our whole lifetime. Ultimately science discovered that, in fact, with certain behaviors we can develop new brain cells, as well as build and strengthen the connections between these brain cells. This is known as *neuroplasticity.*

Another interesting fact is that our brains develop with a strong negative bias toward rumination and vigilance from an area called the *amygdala.* This area worries about past events and focuses on potential problems in future events. Many people refer to this as *monkey brain.* One of the significant issues we see when our brain follows this path is that chemical changes create significant stress. This leads to significant problems in many areas of the body and processes, some of which we have already mentioned. This is where the neuroplasticity comes in. By practicing the *mindful* techniques, as well as the physical activity and nutrition we will discuss later, you can develop more brain cells with much stronger connections. This happens in the parts of the brain that help to calm your mind,  and which also make many significant changes in the biochemistry and physiology of other parts of your body. This change in your brain alters areas like your microbiome, as well as some molecules from your endocrine system, such as cortisol. And we will learn later that exercise or *movement* also produces a chemical that helps grow brain cells.

So, as you can see from our brief review already, the connections and interactions of the various parts and systems in our bodies are very complex and intricate. I refer to this beautiful interaction as the *vibrant synergy* of interconnection of all of our systems. Let me assure you that you don't have to understand or study any of this portion of material. It's great to know, but having a deep understanding of the science is not required. This *workbook* is laid out in such a way that anyone can follow the simple prompts each day. We will slowly lay out information in three areas each day.

Consider this important point. As we go through life, most things around us may come or go, or be replaced as needed. I'm referring to objects like houses, cars, and other possessions. In addition, interests, friends, jobs, taste in music, foods we prefer— all of these things can change many times.

Although it may not be a pleasant consideration, this idea even applies to the people we know and love, including family. They all can, and will, move into and out of our lives over time. This could be birth or death or many other reasons. There are two things with you from the beginning to the end of your life. One is your physical body. The other is your mind. Both of these have to last, as well as possible, as long as you are here. For a moment, let's consider what you might do differently with the possessions above if they had to last your lifetime. Now with that consideration in mind, wouldn't it be wise to take as much care and interest in maintaining the only vessel we have in life as well or even better than the individual relationships and the many possessions listed above?

An analogy I like is this. The vessel you will occupy in life would be best treated as your masterpiece! Much like Pablo Picasso created his masterpieces — one canvas, one paintbrush, and picking colors one stroke at a time. This occurred minute to minute and day to day. Each day he focused on only that portion of work, but over time it came together as a masterpiece for the ages.

You will be learning simple techniques that when you apply them day after day, time after time, choosing the "canvas, brush, and colors" you want, *you* will become your *masterpiece*. You will pick the techniques that fit with your life, wishes, and tastes. This is your journey! No two journeys are identical. I do encourage you to check into each technique and consider learning something about it. Techniques are like a brush or a jar of paint in Picasso's paint kit. Some may be used more often, but if things change for whatever reason, you will have more choices and skills that you can use if needed.

Each day you will focus on three areas:
1. Movement
2. Optimal Fuel
3. Being

## Preview / Preparation

1. This journey is *your* journey! No two journeys are perfectly identical. You will slowly work though this material and gravitate to the portion that speaks to you and feels like it fits best with you.

2. We will focus on *One Day at a Time,* the day that you are currently living. You should review this concept multiple times a day. Over time you will internalize it.

3. Many people focus on their weight, and while that's not an inherently bad thing, it is more helpful to think about improving your total health and well-being. Being overweight is a problem, but in many ways it is but one symptom of a larger imbalance with regard to the interaction between several systems in your body. This may include nutritional problems, various neuroendocrine and other biochemical imbalances, or a lack of appropriate physical activity leading to poor body conditioning, just to mention a few. Stress and certain lifestyle choices, such as smoking, excessive alcohol consumption, drug use or overuse, can all be contributing factors as well. I find it much more helpful to focus on *maximizing* your *nutritional intake* daily than to watching your weight in particular.

4. The good news is that by addressing the three areas of **Movement, Optimal Fuel,** and **Being** each day, we can readjust these issues over time into a balance that corrects many of these problems. Look back at the selected metabolic problems we discussed that contribute to development of many chronic problems for us. There are some common connections in each of the above three daily areas of focus. By working daily in each of these three areas, we can improve on several common issues.

5. *Movement* is a very broad category. We will address this every day. What you choose to do depends on various factors, including interests, age, fitness level, and health status. The salient point is that you will start exactly where you are. If you have any health issues or other concerns, you will need to get advice from your physician on what is appropriate from a medical standpoint for you. You should start where you are, and safely progress from there as you can. My personal movement program has been largely walking, and this has been very successful for me. Again, each person starts where they are. It is good to introduce some variety. As you can see from our limited review of problems that can develop in the body, Movement not only benefits your musculoskeletal system,

*movement ?*

but additionally has positive effects on the brain, cardiovascular system, mental state, immune system, and many other biochemical and physiological aspects of your body's total health and well-being.

6. *Optimal Fuel* is the second category that we will address every day. This again is an area where we will start slowly and layer in new information day after day. This will be a learning process, but we will help you navigate your way. As we mentioned with Movement above, you will be exposed to many concepts and choices and ultimately you will choose what fits you best for the journey that you desire. Again, our paradigm is not to focus on what you have to deny yourself each day. You want the focus to be on providing the best fuel possible to power the only physical body that I will have to live in my entire life. I want to fuel it up to the best degree possible for my own health and well-being.

7. *Being.* The human brain has evolved such that it has a strong negative bias to alert us to problems potentially in our future. The brain also spends a significant amount of time ruminating about past events that concern us. The problem for us is that this action from the brain creates changes that increase not only our stress response locally, but over time can create significant negative results in other systems and organs in our body. The good news is that you will learn many techniques to use to help you deal with these negative events, which all of us experience from time to time. The results of these techniques are dose-dependent. To illustrate this concept, imagine a person who does arm curls every day with a barbell, but just with their left arm. Over time that left bicep will be larger and stronger than their right bicep. Slowly over time these Being techniques will be helping you learn to improve your awareness of being in the current moment. This creates a myriad of positive effects for your health and well-being. It also has a vibrant synergistic effect with the changes you are making in the other two areas. Over time these techniques become your way of being and not just something you are doing on occasion. You are building a calming oasis in the relaxation portion of the brain, which is totally portable and always available for you anytime you need it.

8. It is advisable that you *journal* each day if possible. Some of the techniques we will be discussing specifically include journaling. Also, it is important to record and review what is working for you and what is not. It is important to have a plan each day with regard to all three areas. Preparation is very helpful to decrease having unexpected events create challenges that increase the probability that you will fall off your plan.

9. You will want to focus on each day as it comes. Everyone has long-term goals.

   The people who are most successful in reaching their ultimate goals learn to reward themselves every day. They take satisfaction in realizing smaller chunks of progress (that is, taking little steps closer to their ultimate goal). We should all learn to appreciate these smaller chunks of progress in movement in the right direction. This is why we say, "Follow your plan to success just today!" This is the way Navy Seals accomplish massive missions so successfully. They focus on small chunks of the process, done well, leading in the right direction; and they mentally reward themselves for this. You will want to remember that each day.

10. This is *your* journey, and it is unique to *you*. We are honored you are allowing us to play a small part in your effort to **Becoming Optimal You!**

    *One Day at a Time.*

# PROLOGUE

This book contains important and powerful information.
The more you follow these suggestions, the more
positive the effect will be.

❀

You could focus on each day's information for
more time before proceeding.

❀

You may decide to spend two days on each day's material
before you proceed, or you could work straight through
and then do it again.

❀

You will notice much repetition, and this is by design.
The more you work on something the more
ingrained it becomes.

❀

Repeated behaviors become **habits**, and repeated habits
can become **traits**.

❀

I encourage you to **journal**, each day, your thoughts, plans,
or issues that come up in each of your three focus areas:
**Movement, Optimal Fuel, and Being**.

❀

Preparation and planning are key to success.

❀

Your journey is your journey.

❀

Live one day at a time!

# DAY 1

*"The best thing about the future is that
it comes one day at a time"*

—Abraham Lincoln

## Movement:

1. Each day, you should incorporate movement.

2. Live life one day at a time!

3. It is important to be aware of your current level of fitness and health.

4. If you have a question about your appropriate level of movement, I encourage you to talk with your healthcare provider.

5. Walking is an excellent activity for a high percentage of people. My personal journey began with walking, and it continues to be over 90 percent of my movement program.

6. I encourage you to keep a **journal** with some ideas and possible choices that speak to you for your movement.

7. Remember, you are looking to increase movement across the day, so it shouldn't require a huge block of time in any portion of your day.

8. Formal exercise or workout times are fine but don't negate the importance of small additions of movement such as bending or stretching while doing all living activities.

## Optimal Fuel:

1. It is wise to consume your nutrition over a fixed amount of time and during the same window each day.

2. The above window could be 10 or 12 hours.

3. This is not a requirement, but there is research that points to an increase in loss of body fat and possible increased longevity for those who follow this regimen. Again, this is not a requirement, but I present it as an additional tool for your consideration.

4. Drink a tall glass of water at the beginning of each meal.

5. It is best to eat three meals per day with two healthy snacks between the meals.

6. Avoid processed sugars and carbohydrates as much as possible.

7. Most pre-packed and manufactured meals contain excessive amounts of simple sugars. They can cause wild swings in blood sugar levels that create problematic hormonal and negative physiological changes in the body.

8. In addition to three meals per day, it is a good idea to have a small, healthy snack between meals (two snacks per day).

**9.** Examples of healthy snacks include:
   a. A small handful of nuts
   b. Carrots or celery and small amount of nut butter
   c. A small apple or banana with nut butter

**10.** Eat slowly, putting your fork or spoon down while chewing.

**11.** Chew more frequently than in the past.

**12.** Preparation and preplanning are very important to help decrease episodes of hunger and binge eating.

**13.** **Journal** any thoughts and plans that may come to you regarding the above **Optimal Fuel** suggestions.

**14.** Over the course of this book, we will be layering information each day. There will be repetition, and this is by design. The goal is to slowly assimilate the nutritional information that speaks to you as we build your personal journey one day at a time.

## Being:

### WHY LIST

a. It is important to spend some time determining your **Why List** for your desire to change your life.

b. Pick out the top three to five Whys.

c. Write these reasons down three times slowly.

d. Write them one more time slowly and read them out loud to yourself as you write them.

e. Now, read them out loud to yourself two more times and, each time, linger on each for at least 30 seconds. In your mind's eye, feel the emotional connection between this **Why** and your desire to make positive changes. Feel the joy, love, or whatever positive emotion this creates for you.

f. You should consider doing this activity every day. In addition, you may want to repeat it at other times of the day as time and your environment allow. Many of the techniques you will learn in the **Being** section are valuable tools that are very helpful to do during your formal set-aside time for such activities. Over the long haul, as it becomes part of your being rather than just something you do on occasion, the vibrant synergy of these techniques will begin to make powerful changes in your life.

## BREATHING EXERCISE:

a. This activity is a part of mindfulness or meditation.

b. If you already practice this, you have a head start. These instructions will help those who have never meditated.

c. The simple explanation, for now, is to practice concentrating on a focus point in the here and now.

d. Decide if you want to either focus on the sensation of your breath or on a mantra, which is a word or phrase you say to yourself with each exhalation or inhalation. It is your choice to make. This choice is your anchor during meditation or breathing exercises.

e. A mantra could be a religious term like Jesus, Buddha, Mother Mary, or God is love, or the universe.

f. The point of the breathing exercise is to practice keeping our mind in the present moment.

g. Our mind develops with a heavy negative bias. This is a protective mechanism for survival. That is the reason our mind ruminates about events in the past and worries about potential bad future events.

h. Each time our mind wanders from our focus, we will nonjudgmentally recognize that and gently bring it back to our breathing anchor.

i. This activity, over time, helps us stay in the moment and helps us deal with the challenges of life much more effectively.

j. Staying in the moment helps create many positive biochemical and physiological changes in our body which have positive effects on our level of joy, health, and even longevity!

### Breathing Meditation Instruction:

1. Set alarm for five to seven minutes.

2. Sit comfortably.

3. Relax your muscles and take a couple deep breaths.

4. Close your eyes.

5. Focus on your natural breathing using your chosen focus method.

6. Each time your mind wanders, bring it back gently and nonjudgmentally.

7. Continue until your time is up.

---

*Positive effects from this breathing exercise are dose-dependent. A weightlifter doing arm curls with a dumbbell each day to build muscle is very analogous. The more practice, the more muscle enlargement or, with meditation, stronger connections between neurons develop in the calming center of the brain. This creates significant health and well-being benefits.*

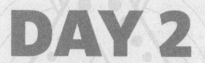

# DAY 2

*"Just keep moving forward, one day at a time. The view from the top of the climb is worth it!"*

—Anonymous

# Movement:

1. Initiate your movement plan for the day.

2. Continually assess the appropriateness of your plan with regard to your current health and fitness level.

3. Focus on today's activity.

4. If there is something that you really enjoy doing, that will be a bonus.

5. For many people, walking is an excellent activity.

6. I encourage you to **journal** thoughts, ideas, and plans for your movement program.

# Optimal Fuel:

Today we will give an outline of three general categories of high quality, nutritionally dense foods that we should eat as much as possible to provide the best fuel for our body to run on. We will also list a couple of categories that are nutritionally lacking and contain many empty calories and/or compounds that create significant health and wellness problems.

## General Rules:

1. It is best to pick a window of 10 to 12 hours each day that you consume all your nutrition. This is not a hard requirement, but it can be helpful.

2. Drink a tall glass of water at the beginning of each meal.

3. Eat slowly and chew more times than you normally would in the past. Savor the aroma, flavor, and the texture of the food as you chew and swallow.

4. Eat until satisfied but do not stuff yourself.

5. Follow the three **do** sections and two **avoid** sections below as closely as possible.

6. A small snack between meals is acceptable.

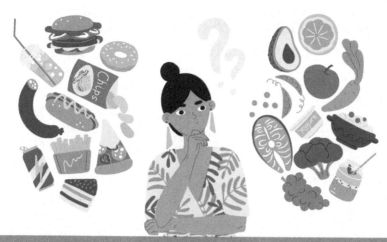

## Do Lists:

### Eat Complex Carbohydrates:

1. You should have several servings of vegetables and fruits daily. You should choose from several varieties and try to eat the "rainbow of color" daily. Fresh or frozen are best to consume.

2. Eat various types of beans, lentils, and peas.

3. Eat nuts and seeds such as sunflower, chia, or flax seeds. Nuts, including walnuts, cashews, pistachios and others, are very healthy.

4. Whole grains should be consumed regularly. Examples include chickpeas, hummus, brown rice, quinoa, steel cut oats, millets, barley, rye, and buckwheat.

5. Eat sweet potatoes.

### Eat Quality Protein:

1. Any fish is good. Wild caught salmon, sardines, mackerel, and anchovies are also excellent sources of Omega-3 fats as well as high quality protein.

2. Lean beef (limit one or two servings per week)

3. Various seeds and nuts

4. A variety of beans, lentils, and peas

5. Chicken or turkey (do not consume skin)

6. Greek yogurt

7. Tofu

8. Kefir

9. Pork loin

10. Eggs

### Eat Nourishing Fats:

1. Avocado

2. Olives and in addition you should cook in extra-virgin olive oil

3. Dark chocolate (over 70 percent cocoa)

4. Nuts, seeds, and nut butter

5. Oily fish like wild caught salmon, sardines, mackerel, and anchovies

## Avoid

**Solid Fats:**

1. Butter, margarine, and cream

2. Bacon

3. All processed meats including hots dogs, salami, and lunchmeat

4. Ribs

5. Steak fat

6. Chicken or turkey skin

7. Lard

8. Hydrogenated oils and vegetable oils

**Simple Carbohydrates:**

1. Avoid breads other than whole grain

2. Avoid pasta unless made from chickpeas, lentils, edamame, or beans

3. Simple sugars (this includes fruit juices and soda pop)

4. White rice

5. Potatoes

6. Alcohol, except the occasional glass of red wine

7. Avoid flour, including cereals, cakes, and cookies

8. As much as possible, avoid foods that have been refined, processed, or manufactured

## Final Tips

1. Focus on the quality of nutrition that you consume every day.

2. Do not focus on cutting back calories. Focus on cutting back consumption of low nutritional-content foods. Work to increase the quality of nutrition in each of your meals.

3. Be sure to drink enough fluids every day. Water, tea, and coffee would be the healthiest. By putting lemon in your water or tea you are increasing your antioxidant consumption. Tea, especially green tea, as well as coffee are already high in antioxidants. This helps boost your immune system significantly.

4. We recommend Stevia as a low-calorie sweetener for your beverages, if needed.

5. Use of turmeric, ginger, cinnamon, garlic, paprika, parsley, and many other spices are very healthy and should be used freely to taste.

6. Remember, 70–80 percent or more of the food you consume each

meal should be plant-based. I will mention here that the science does indicate that a plant-based diet is the healthiest. Many people choose to consume some animal-based foods and I, also, choose to do that on a limited basis. This program, while not perfect, is very healthy if followed closely.

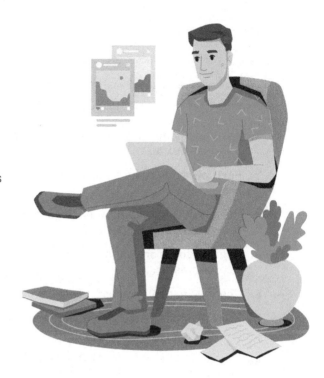

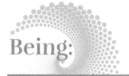

Being:

**WHY LIST**

a. Slowly write your **Why List**.

b. As you write each entry, linger slowly over it for 20–30 seconds.

c. With eyes closed and in your mind's eye, feel the connection and emotion that this particular **Why List** elicits in you.

d. Go through this at least three times.

e. As you continue to do this daily, over time you are building neural synapses in the calming part of the brain. This will help you as you revisit these important reasons during times of stress or lower motivation.

f. Stress, anxiety, and even boredom can increase the probability that you will enlist behaviors that are counterproductive to your ability to make significant positive changes to unhealthy behaviors.

## MEDITATION/BREATHING EXERCISE:

**a.** Assume a comfortable position, set timer, and push button.

**b.** Feel your feet on the ground and your buttock on your chair.

**c.** Quickly scan your body, then begin to take a couple slow and deep breaths.

**d.** Begin to focus on your anchor attached to your breaths.

**e.** Continue to gently focus on anchor.

**f.** You will notice, possibly multiple times, that your mind wanders. This is normal and natural.

**g.** Your goal is to, upon noticing the change, gently and nonjudgmentally pull your focus back to your anchor.

**h.** Continue until time is up.

**i.** This activity, over time, helps us stay in the moment and helps us deal with the challenges of life much more effectively.

**j.** Again, remember that, over time, you are building and connecting actual brain cells in the calming portion of the brain, as well as stronger connections between neurons to more effectively counteract negative effects of stress, not only on the brain, but on many other important areas of the body.

### Breathing Meditation Instruction:

1. Set alarm for five to seven minutes.

2. Sit comfortably.

3. Relax your muscles and take a couple deep breaths.

4. Close your eyes.

5. Focus on your natural breathing using your chosen focus method.

6. Each time your mind wanders, bring it back gently and nonjudgmentally.

7. Continue until your time is up.

---

*Positive effects from this breathing exercise are dose-dependent. A weightlifter doing arm curls with a dumbbell each day to build muscle is very analogous. The more practice, the more muscle enlargement or, with meditation, stronger connections between neurons develop in the calming center of the brain. This creates significant health and well-being benefits.*

# DAY 3

"The journey of 1,000 miles begins
with the first step."

—Lao Tzu

# Movement:

1. Movement is not just the time you are at the gym or when you walk around the block.

2. The above actions are great, but there are many creative ways you can add to your movement.

3. One interesting finding is the people who live in the Blue Zones (areas of the world that have high numbers of people living over 100 years) tend to move more with regular activity throughout the day by gardening, cleaning, chores, and other activities of daily living.

4. Finding movement in many different activities is a good strategy. This does not mean forget the gym or your daily dog walk. It does mean that the value of your movement program is from the sum total of movement for the day.

5. If you go to the market, you could walk up and down all the aisles a few times more than would be required just to shop. If you are in inclement weather states in winter, you can find warm, safe aisles to walk in and clean, safe restrooms in most major stores. Parking further away from stores or other destinations in good weather and safe areas is another good strategy.

6. If watching television, you could get up and walk door-to-door during commercial breaks. I have occasionally paced back and forth in the room as I watch a program.

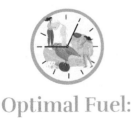

## Optimal Fuel:

1. Pick your window of time to eat.

2. Eat three meals per day and two snacks between meals.

3. Drink a tall glass of water at beginning of your meal.

4. Eat slowly.

5. Daily: **Eat Rainbows of Color** of fruits and vegetables to maximize many nutrients.

6. Whole grains are very nutritious.

## Sample Healthy Meals:

### Breakfast:

Three eggs but only one yolk, scrambled or omelet. Add in chopped spinach, onions, tomato, colored peppers, mushrooms, milled flax seed, and a small amount feta cheese. Cook in olive oil and garlic, salt and pepper to taste. Add various fruit.

### Lunch:

Diverse greens salad, carrots, celery, cucumber, mushrooms, colored peppers, tomato, onion, hummus and milled flax seeds. Dressing of mixed olive oil, balsamic vinegar, and apple cider vinegar. Choice of protein on salad of:

a) Chicken; grilled or baked; season to taste

b) Tofu

c) Beans, quinoa, or lentils

d) Seafood of salmon, tuna, sardines, mackerel, oysters, or shrimp

### Dinner:

In crock pot, slow cook:

1. Various beans, mixed

2. Broth, either vegetable, bone, or chicken

3. Various mixed vegetables, fresh or frozen

4. Add spices to taste

5. This is easy to make enough for additional meals.

### Dessert:

Plain Greek yogurt; add frozen berries

### Beverages:

1. Water; add lemon for taste and antioxidants

2. Tea, green, or other

3. Coffee, also high in antioxidants

# Being:

## WHY LIST

a. Write your list slowly three times.

b. Linger on each reason for 20–30 seconds each time, and, in your mind's eye, appreciate and feel the love and/or the importance each reason has for you.

c. I encourage you, at other times of the day when the opportunity arises, to think about the items on the list or do the same thing in your mind. Each time you do this, you are building synapses stronger and increasing numbers and sizes of neurons in the appropriate calming part of the brain. This will help you to counteract the negative impact when stress or other issues tempt you to revert to old ways. When feeling the pull of possibly making poor behavior choices, you will be able to visualize these positive motivating **Whys** and rest with them internally to counteract the pull of your negative triggers.

d. If you do backslide, do not fret. Each day is a new day, and you only need to concentrate on right here, right now.

## MEDITATION/ BREATHING EXERCISE:

a. Continue to practice this at least five minutes per day.

b. If you have time during the day, you can do this again, even with eyes open, if needed.

c. This also is something you can do at other times of the day when you have a moment, and this activity comes to mind. Over time, this is what you want to do so as to seamlessly integrate these techniques into your daily activities. This is when you transform from these being techniques that you do to it becoming your way of being. Many positive benefits will manifest in your life when you get to this state of being.

### Breathing Meditation Instruction:

1. Set alarm for five to seven minutes.
2. Sit comfortably.
3. Relax your muscles and take a couple deep breaths.
4. Close your eyes.
5. Focus on your natural breathing using your chosen focus method.
6. Each time your mind wanders, bring it back gently and nonjudgmentally.
7. Continue until your time is up.

*Positive effects from this breathing exercise are dose-dependent. A weightlifter doing arm curls with a dumbbell each day to build muscle is very analogous. The more practice, the more muscle enlargement or, with meditation, stronger connections between neurons develop in the calming center of the brain. This creates significant health and well-being benefits.*

# DAY 4

*"It's not just about what you are eating, it's also about what's eating you!"*

—Anonymous

*I will focus just on today. Part of my goal for today is to keep my attention on whatever **movement** I plan for this day. I will be attentive, just for today, to the quality of the **fuel** that I put into the only vessel I will ever have to exist in. Finally, I will study, practice, and repeat the techniques that will help me develop resilience to life's challenges and awareness of living in the moment. This will also help me to spend much less time ruminating about past events and worrying about potential future negative events. I will live one day at a time.*

## Movement:

1. Write down a general movement in today's plan.

2. It's good to take a moment at the beginning of your day to consider how your movement plan is progressing.

3. Planning and preparation are key in all three areas.

4. Is what you are doing feeling like something you enjoy?

5. Do things that speak to your heart.

6. Are there ways I can combine these other daily activities? Examples might be during work, when you get up from your desk, stretch and walk some steps to the hall or around your room.

7. Are there steps you can be taking even at break time?

8. When parking for errands, park farther away.

9. Focus on varied moving activities.

10. I will look for opportunities to do some stretching.

11. I will look for ways to incorporate resistance in my exercise.

12. Are there stairs that I can safely go up and down for tolerance building?

13. I will journal and plan my movement for this day.

14. Find enjoyable movement today!

## Optimal Fuel:

**1.** I will plan in advance what my meal plan will look like.

**2.** I will have snacks available to prevent unplanned binging should triggers for unwanted hunger or bad food choices occur.

**3.** I will remember to have available food choices from the **Do Choose** section to maximize the quality and diversity of nutrients just for this day.

**4.** I will remember that if I'm traveling and run short on healthy food, it is often easier to get healthier choices by going to a grocery store as opposed to fast food restaurants. One can pick up a yogurt, a package of salmon or tuna, or grilled chicken in the deli. They often have healthy salad choices near the deli. There is also a broad choice of fruits and vegetables in the produce area.

**5.** It is wise to have disposable cutlery and plates and napkins in your vehicle for such urgent situations.

### Typical Meals:

| Breakfast: | Good protein/good fat/complex carbohydrates | |
|---|---|---|
| **Snack:** | Protein/fat/carb | at least two of the three |
| **Lunch:** | Protein/fat/carb | all three |
| **Snack:** | Protein/fat/carb | at least two of the three |
| **Dinner:** | Protein/fat/carb | all three |

### Example Breakfast:

1. **Steel cut oats 1/4 – 1/3 cup**

2. **Cinnamon powder**

3. **Stevia to sweeten, if preferred**

4. **Chia seeds**

5. **Add mixed fruit** to your taste after heating Instructions:

Let it soak in water overnight; put in microwave for approximately two minutes. Enjoy!

———

*Each day remember to pick a variety of fruits and vegetables with an emphasis on various colors. This denotes different nutrients which are needed to keep you healthy. They are not only important for your physical well-being, but they can play a significant part in your emotional state, your cognitive abilities, as well as your immune system which increases your ability to fight outside pathogens as well as mutations that can occur in your body. These mutations can lead to various disease states including cancers of many types.*

## Being:

**WHY LIST**

**a.** Write your "why change inventory" at least three times slowly and linger on each one with closed eyes. Visualize each one as you see and feel each internally. Allow yourself to feel the warmth and love each gives you. Sense how important each is to you.

**b.** Practice your meditative breathing exercise.

A good habit to develop is to **journal** each day about what you've learned. Note what touches or speaks to your heart. You may want to emphasize that.

**a.** Each day, repeat the activities above silently and verbally any time they come to mind. This can be sitting at your desk, walking down the hallway, or walking to your car after work. By doing this, you are strengthening the synapsis between neurons in the calming area each time you bring your attention back to memories, issues, or people who are so meaningful to you. Each time you practice, you are nourishing your physical brain and emotional mind in a way that will, over time, help you handle stress against life's challenges. This is known as building resilience. We will go further into this in a bit. For now, keep practicing and building your Becoming Optimal You, one day at a time.

# DAY 5

*"Everybody is looking for instant success, but it doesn't work that way. You build a successful life one day at a time."*

—Abraham Lincoln

## *Movement, Optimal Fuel, Being—just today*

# Movement:

1. Do I start my day with a plan?

2. Do I stretch and warm up appropriately?

3. Am I doing something that I enjoy?

4. Is this something I can do with others? This could build community and bonding, as well as increase the enjoyment and connectivity. Thus, this will increase probability of continuing my activity.

5. I will remember that any additional movement at any time today is part of strengthening my muscles, bones, ligaments and my cardiovascular system. I am also having positive effects on higher levels of neurotransmitters that help my mental state, as well increasing the numbers, size, and connections of neurons in the calming centers of my brain. I am also lowering my risk for degenerative brain disorders including Alzheimer's. I am having a positive effect on many physiological and biochemical reactions in my body, which lowers my risk for many chronic diseases, as well as many types of cancer.

6. Remember, the result of my activity today is additive with every other day in improving my health and well-being.

7. My effort today is my only focus today. If I don't have a large block of time, I will do what I can, when I can.

8. I will **journal** my movement plan.

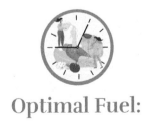

# Optimal Fuel:

1. I will remember that preparation and planning are very helpful to be successful in my efforts today.

2. I will **journal** my plan.

3. I am focusing on just today.

4. I will have a plan for consumption of optimal nutrition today.

5. I will try to learn something new each day about **Optimal**

**Fuel** to consume for my health and well-being.

**6.** As part of my plan to be more mindful in all aspects of my life, I will try to avoid eating while watching or listening to something else.

**7.** I will be grateful and express it prior to nutrition consumption.

**8.** I will chew slowly, put down my utensils, enjoy the taste, aroma, and physical sensation of my food.

**9.** I will be more mindful.

---

**IDEAL FOR HEALTHY EATING:**
- ✓ Three meals per day
- ✓ Two snacks per day
- ✓ Drink a tall glass of water at beginning of meal.

---

## Sample Meals:

**Typical Breakfast:**

Three eggs, but only one yolk, omelet or scrambled; add in chopped spinach, tomatoes, mushrooms, multicolored peppers, and onion. Cook in olive oil, add garlic, flax seeds, salt, pepper. Dessert: mixed fruit.

**Typical Lunch:**

Greens/salad with multicolored veggies added.
  *Protein — chicken, fish or tofu*

**Dressing:** I mix balsamic/apple cider/wine vinegar. Also, flax seeds and feta.

**Dessert:** Various fruits with plain Greek yogurt; 100 percent cocoa and chia seeds.

**Typical Dinner Examples:**

1. Pasta made of whole grain chickpeas, lentils, black beans or edamame. I make sauce from two cans diced tomatoes, one small can tomato paste with garlic salt, oregano to taste, and olive oil

2. Bean Soup — mix various beans with bone or chicken broth. Add mixed frozen veggies; spices to taste.

3. Baked or broiled fish or chicken. Side: broccoli, green beans, whole grain.
Dessert: various fruits

**Dessert:**

Green tea, Stevia to sweeten if needed

Coffee or water

Drink a glass of water before meals and after most bites

**Healthy Snack Options:**

Handful of nuts

Carrots or celery with peanut butter

Apple or banana with or without peanut butter

Handful of berries/other fruit

# Being:

1. *You will want to have a plan for practicing your Being techniques.*

2. *It will be helpful to journal about your experiences and plans for your Being portion of your program.*

3. *We will be layering in multiple techniques in the course of this program. You are encouraged to work with them, and, ultimately, there may be some that speak more to your personal likes or that touch you in such a way as to enhance your personal journey to living more mindfully. You may use some more than others if you choose. This is your journey. The goal is to use what we have learned through neuroscience to make positive changes in your brain that will help you be more self-aware and live more mindfully. By doing so, you will greatly improve your health, wellness, and general well-being. You will not only be making tremendous improvements in your life, but you will be having a much more positive impact on those you love, as well as all you come in contact with.*

## WHY LIST

1. Continue to repeat your **Why** List.

2. During the day when you have the opportunity, it will be helpful to internally visualize each **Why**. Linger on each one a bit and silently say each to yourself. Feel the emotion that each evokes.

3. This can be done with eyes open at your desk, and it is a short break from your daily activity. No one need be aware.

4. Continue to work, write, and repeat this activity during your formal meditative time.

5. You may also do this prior to meals or other times you may feel a pull toward reverting to previous unhealthy behavior.

## MEDITATION:

1. Continue as described in formal meditative time.

2. Adjust and increase time as you feel comfortable.

3. This also can be repeated many times a day with eyes open if needed for relaxation and practice.

4. The more you practice, the more you will come to appreciate the sense of calm and contentment you feel soon after dropping into your cocoon of just being. It is portable and can be with you anytime, anywhere.

# DAY 6

*"Live one day at a time and
make it a masterpiece."*

—Dale West

*Focus on just this day. Today starts with me right here, right now, just as I am. I will have a plan for today, and I will follow my plan. I will **journal** my plan.*

*I remember that the longest journey started with the first step. This is my journey. I will learn, practice, and ultimately utilize the techniques that speak to me and feel like a natural fit for my journey.*

## Movement:

1. I will do the movement today that is appropriate for my fitness level.

2. I will do movement today that speaks to me with enjoyment and contentment.

3. I will visualize that, as I move, I am nourishing my muscles, bones, ligaments, and cardiovascular system.

4. My movement will nourish my brain.

5. I will consider journaling on my movement today.

6. I will attempt to vary my program when needed to keep it fresh.

7. I will look for opportunities to do movement with friends or a likeminded group to add interest and help develop a sense of community. There are many studies showing the wellness benefits of connection and relationships with others.

## Optimal Fuel:

1. Today I will give my body the best nourishment possible.

2. I will pick a variety of foods that will satisfy my taste palate while also providing an array of nutrients which nourish my body and mind to the maximum degree possible.

3. Protein, fiber, healthy fats, and complex carbohydrates.

4. I will consume less processed food.

5. Consider journaling on your plan for today and the challenges you expect.

**PEARLS**

**Protein sources for weight loss:**

1. Black beans
2. Lima beans
3. Corn
4. Salmon
5. Broccoli
6. Cauliflower
7. Eggs
8. Chicken
9. Bran oats

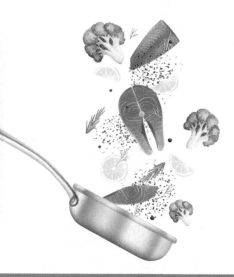

## Sample Meals:

**Typical Breakfast:**

Three eggs, but only one yolk, omelet or scrambled; add in chopped spinach, tomatoes, mushrooms, multicolored peppers, and onion. Cook in olive oil and add garlic, flax seeds, salt, and pepper. Dessert: mixed fruit.

**Typical Lunch:**

Greens/salad with multicolored veggies added.
*Protein — chicken, fish or tofu*

**Dressing:** I mix balsamic/apple cider/ wine vinegar. Also, flax seeds and feta.

**Dessert:** Various fruits with plain Greek yogurt;

100 percent cocoa and chia seeds.

**Typical Dinner Examples:**

1. Pasta made of whole grain chickpeas, lentils, black beans or edamame. I make sauce from two cans diced tomatoes, one small can tomato paste with garlic salt, oregano to taste, and olive oil

2. Bean Soup — mix various beans with bone or chicken broth. Add mixed frozen veggies; spices to taste.

3. Baked or broiled fish or chicken. Side: broccoli,

green beans, whole grain.
Dessert: various fruit

**Dessert:**

Green tea, Stevia to sweeten if needed

Coffee or water

Drink a glass of water before meals and after most bites

**Healthy Snack Options:**

Handful of nuts

Carrots or celery with peanut butter

Apple or banana with or without peanut butter

Handful of berries/ other fruit

# Being:

## WHY LIST

1. Continue to repeat your **Why List**, writing, visualizing, and lingering on each **Why** is very powerful. You are growing neurons and strengthening the synapse between them each time you do this. The more you do this, the more positive the effect will be on the brain, similar to the bicep that is repeatedly exercised by doing curls with a dumbbell. In this instance, these increased positive connections will be an easily accessible counterweight that we will use during regular meditation to help counterbalance triggers for unwanted behaviors. We will discuss this in a bit but, for now, know that these repeated exercises will be very helpful for you as we progress.

2. It will be helpful, during your day when you have the opportunity, to internally visualize each Why. Linger on each one a bit and silently say each to yourself. Feel the emotion that each evokes.

3. This can be done with eyes open at your desk, and it is a short break from your daily activity. No one need be aware.

4. Continue to work, write, and repeat this activity during your formal meditative time.

5. You may also do this prior to meals or other times you may feel a pull toward reverting to previous unhealthy behavior.

## MEDITATION:

1. Continue as described in formal meditative time.

2. Adjust and increase time as you feel comfortable.

3. This also can be repeated many times a day with eyes open if needed for relaxation and practice.

4. Sit comfortably. Take a couple slow deep breaths.

5. Feel your shoulders relax.

6. Feel your buttocks on your chair and your feet on the ground.

7. Allow your attention to go to your meditation anchor.

8. When your mind wanders, as it normally will, in a gentle and nonjudgmental way, bring your attention back to the anchor. You may repeat that many times.

9. Be patient with yourself. This can feel uncomfortable and, often, people can't decide if they are doing it correctly. It is so worth the effort to continue doing this activity. The benefits for you over time are vast and profound. It is absolutely free. It is completely portable.

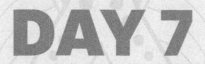

# DAY 7

"*Because you are alive,
everything is possible.*"

—Thich Nhat Hanh

*I begin today just as I am. Right here, right now. Today I will nourish the only body and mind I will ever have to the best of my ability. I will do this not only for myself and my loved ones, but for the betterment of all mankind. Just for today, I focus on **Movement**, **Optimal Fuel**, and **Being**.*

# Movement:

1. I will continue my movement program.

2. I will continue to do what is safe and enjoyable for me.

3. I will look for opportunities to connect my movement with other healthy behaviors to maximize the value of the time I spend in this activity. An example would be to spend time focusing on some meditative **Being** exercises while doing my movement.

4. When possible, I will do some of my movement with others which helps build community.

5. Examples of the above steps could be fundraising or door-to-door activities to help others in need. There are many ways to do good for others while also increasing my movement for that day.

# Optimal Fuel:

1. I will continue to focus on consuming the best nutrition possible today to keep my body and mind as healthy as possible.

2. I will learn something new each day about foods and nutrients that are most beneficial for my health and well-being.

3. I will strive to plan my eating for the day prior to it starting. This will help me avoid hunger and stress, which may increase bad decisions in nutritional and behavioral choices.

4. I will plan my meals in advance to whatever degree possible.

5. I will journal about my Optimal Fuel program.

6. I will consume a broad array of foods each day to maximize my exposure to needed nutrients.

7. I will consume foods as close to their natural state as possible.

**NUTRITIONAL PEARL**

**QUESTION:**
**What do antioxidants do?**

**Answer:** *They help prevent cellular damage, which can lead to serious chronic diseases such as many cancers, diabetes, heart disease, dementia, and many others. The damage from oxidation can advance aging. The process of oxidation is just like the iron portion under a bridge crossing when it becomes covered in rust. That is an oxidative process and causes damage and possible weakening of the bridge.*

**Plants that are high in antioxidants:**

1. Leafy greens
2. Berries of all types
3. Spices including, but not limited to: Rosemary, Sage, Oregano, Turmeric, and Paprika
4. Beans
5. Artichokes
6. Prunes
7. Raw garlic
8. Dark chocolate
9. Grapes; all colors

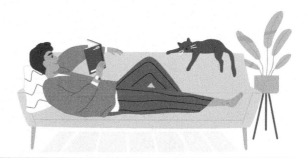

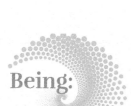

Being:

**WHY LIST**

1. Repeat this list each day.

2. This is also something you can bring to mind and visualize when you have down time at work, relaxation time, or while during chores. Just repeat your **Why List** silently and linger on each one for at least 20 seconds or more. Feel the emotion that each **Why** item evokes in you! Feel that positive connection that is strong enough for you to want to make positive changes.

3. You can repeat this daily as you wish and can complete.

## MEDITATION

1. If possible, continue to perform this activity each day.

2. Very slowly, overtime if you wish, you can increase the time per session.

3. As you gain experience, you may decide to do additional short or micro meditation at other times of the day.

4. Each of these practice sessions are additive to the change being made to the connections between neurons in the calming position of your brain. Not only are you making more neurons in these desired areas of the brain, but you are also growing stronger connections. This is the definition of neuroplasticity.

**TRIGGER LIST:**

1. There is some value in writing down the triggers you respond to by doing the negative behaviors that contribute to you being less healthy.

2. I encourage you to write these daily. Then, think about taking your mind to your **Why List** or **meditation** activity when a trigger pops up in order decrease the trigger's effect on your behavior choice at that time.

3. One of the benefits of focusing on and practicing the **Being** techniques is it helps us become more aware of negative feelings and emotions when they come up.

4. In our previous life, we would deal with these negative issues with negative behaviors such as consuming simple sugars, alcohol, drugs, smoke cigarettes, or get emotionally upset in ways that can cause negative physiological changes impacting our health and well-being.

5. Over time, as we become aware of these negative emotions, we can use our **Why List** and our **meditative breathing practice** in positive ways to deal with these negative emotions. Therefore, we prevent the alternative undesired negative trigger behavior. We will go into this further along.

# DAY 8

*"Smile, breath, and go slowly."*

—Thich Nhat Hanh

*This day is like all others; it is the only one we are living in. Right here, right now is all we really have. Just like Pablo Picasso creating his masterpiece, today we are working on our lives. It is the only masterpiece we have to live in. Pablo Picasso used one brush, one color of paint, one canvas, and one stroke at a time. Today is the only time that we can decide the evolution of our masterpiece—right here, right now. Today's choices of **Movement, Optimal Fuel, and Being**.*

## Movement:

1. Just today, choose to do movement that is enjoyable and invigorating for you.

2. Each time you move, you are strengthening your muscles, ligaments, tendons, and joints.

3. Movement helps to develop strong lungs.

4. Exercise increases a chemical known as Brain-derived neurotrophic factor, which is a hormone that helps your body keep a healthy balance. This includes good brain health and decreased risk of diabetes.

5. Movement helps decrease my risk of multiple types of cancer as well as coronary artery disease.

6. Focus just on today with nourishing movement.

7. Plan, monitor, and assess your activity today.

8. I will remember to stretch each day and do some resistance work that is appropriate for my level of fitness.

9. I will journal on my experience, plans, thoughts, and new ideas.

10. I will consider moving to music or dancing while being aware of my movements and the energy that is making its way through my body.

## Optimal Fuel:

**1.** Today I will nourish my body, mind, and spirit with the best fuel possible.

**2.** I will remember this is the ONLY vessel I have to live my life in.

**3.** I will focus just on today.

**4.** I will take a couple of slow, deep breaths at the beginning of each meal and eat slowly.

**5.** I will put down my utensils and savor the flavor, texture, and scent of my food.

**6.** I will hear the chewing of the food.

**7.** While it is not always possible, I will, as often as I can, eat when not doing other things such as looking at my phone, watching television, or generally being distracted from my meal.

**8.** This approach fits in with trying to increase our awareness with what we are doing at any given time along with what physical and/or emotional feelings or messages we are getting. The more we develop this ability, the less likely we are to revert to autopilot behaviors that are counterproductive for our health and well-being. This does not happen overnight. It is part of the process of living more mindfully.

**9.** The process is one meal at a time, one day at a time.

**10.** I will be grateful for the blessing of my food, and I will verbalize it at each meal.

### PEARLS

**a) Why are antioxidants important?**

- They protect against free radicals.

**b) What do free radicals do?**

- They damage cells in the body which leads to many diseases. This cell damage is called oxidation. It is caused by chemical changes in the body from eating processed foods, lack of exercise, aging, some chemicals, and stress.

**c) What are some problems created by this oxidation?**

- This contributes to heart disease, diabetes, dementia, many cancers, early aging, and premature death, to name a few.

**d) What can I do about it?**

- Increase movement as discussed in this program.

- Eat a diet as we discussed in **Optimal Fuel.**

- Decrease negative effects of stress by employing **Being** strategies in our daily lives.

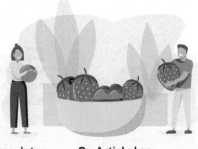

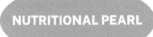

**NUTRITIONAL PEARL**

**More Foods Rich in Antioxidants:**

1. Blueberries
2. Beans
3. Strawberries
4. Kale
5. Dark Chocolate
6. Goji berries
7. Red Cabbage
8. Raspberries
9. Artichokes
10. Pears

# Being:

## WHY LIST

1. Just for today, focus on today.

2. Continue to revisit your **Why List** daily. Each time that you do, you are enlarging the synaptic connections in the brain, which will help to counteract impulses to repeat behaviors that are counter to you becoming the healthiest and best you possible. That is the goal you are striving for.

3. Continue with your breathing exercise for the same reason mentioned before. You are building a stronger core of calm and solitude that is easier to get to the more you practice. Day 9's motivational quote, which follows in tomorrow's plan, says this message very well.

4. Continue reviewing your **Unwanted Behavior Trigger list.**

5. Awareness of potential pitfalls allows you to plan and use the techniques you are learning to counteract triggers when needed.

6. Visualize using your new tools if and when triggers arise.

7. Practice and **journal** on your **Being** tools.

8. Live one day at a time.

9. I am my own master, just like Pablo Picasso created his masterpiece. Each day is one brush, one dip of paint, and one stroke of the hand at a time.

10. I will be grateful that I can move, take nourishment, and be.

11. I will work my **Why List** today.

12. I will practice my meditative breathing today.

13. I will review and prepare for my unwanted behavior list.

# DAY 9

*"Meditation is the ultimate mobile device. You can use it anywhere, anytime  unobtrusively"*
—Sharon Salzberg

*Today is the only day I currently have. I will strive to do the best I can to follow my plan for today. I will continue to journal plans, thoughts, and issues that arise. I will drop into the current moment with my awareness during various times of the day including during **Movement** activities and **Optimal Fuel** activities. Ultimately I will remember there is a vibrant synergy when, on a daily basis, I make an effort to improve myself in each area. You are becoming the Optimal you. You are developing the newer you one day at a time.*

## Movement:

1.  Just for today I will nourish my body, mind, and being with movement.

2.  I will choose movement that I enjoy and that my body, mind, and spirit will respond to with a sense enjoyment and contentment.

3.  Movement will help improve mood and energy.

4.  Movement will help lower risk for several cancers.

5.  I will mix up my activity on occasion to keep it fresh and exciting.

6.  I will consider increasing movement in a manner where I can develop relationships with others and take advantage of the health benefits available to those who have a sense of community and strong relationships with others as they grow older. Group physical activities are a good way to address two positives at one time.

7.  I will attempt to do some resistance exercise, to an appropriate degree, two to three times weekly.

8.  I will stretch and warm up appropriately each day.

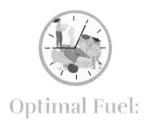

## Optimal Fuel:

1. I will focus on maximizing the value of nutrition I consume today.

2. I will review the categories of nutrition from which I will choose my meals.

3. I will choose a broad array of different colored fruits and vegetables, knowing these colors signify various vitamins and phytonutrients. Together, these will help me maintain the

best health and well-being possible.

**4.** I will minimize the number of manu-factured foods I eat.

**5.** I will look for opportunities to include various high nutrition foods in many of my meals or desserts to diversify and increase the Optimal Fuel value of each meal. Some examples would include flaxseeds or chia seeds. I add these to yogurt with frozen fruit and 100 percent cocoa. I will also add flaxseeds or chia seeds along with cinnamon powder to my steel cut oatmeal. I may also put a dab of Greek yogurt on my oatmeal.

**6.** I will have plans in place for snacks or other issues that might arise on any given day.

**7.** Preparation and forethought are key to success in reaching your goal.

**8.** Your focus is on today!

### THREE HEALTHY BEVERAGES:

**Water with lemon:**

- Detoxifies liver
- Vitamin C helps improve digestive system
- Has anti-inflammatory properties

**Coffee:**

- Reduces risk of Diabetes 2 and Alzheimer's
- Contains powerful antioxidants

**Green Tea:**

- Contains high levels of antioxidants
- Contains Polyphenols, which are anti-inflammatory and anticarcinogenic

## Being:

### WHY LIST

**1.** Today, just focus on today.

**2.** I will practice my breathing meditation exercise daily.

**3.** I will practice visualizing and ingraining my **Why Healthy Behavior list.**

**4.** Each and every day, I will mentally linger on each **Why**, visualize it in my mind's eye, and feel the emotional connection I get from each of my "**Why** make positive change" reasons on my list.

5. Each time I review these tools, I will develop a stronger ability to live the life that I desire, one day at a time.

6. In my daily life, when needed or when I remember to, I will use my tools again and again. This will continue to develop the neurosynaptic connections in the calming centers of my brain, from a thin thread to a broadband superhighway. I will do this practice as many times as I can, each and every day.

7. I will journal on my experiences today as well as on ideas and areas to investigate.

## MEDITATION

1. If possible, I will continue to perform this activity each day.

2. Very slowly over time, if you wish, you can increase the time per session.

3. As you gain experience, you may decide to do additional short or micro meditations at other times of the day.

4. Each of these practice sessions is additive to the change being made to the connections between neurons in the calming control center of your brain.

# DAY 10

*"As long as you are breathing, there is more right with you than wrong with you, no matter what is wrong."*

—Jon Kabat-Zinn

*I will focus just on today. The longest trip still comes down to one step after another. I will strive to stay aware as this day unfolds moment by moment. I will train my mind to spend less time ruminating about negative past events or fretting about potential future problems. By following my* **Movement,** **Optimal Fuel,** *and* **Being** *programs, I am creating an environment where I will become the* **Optimal Me.** *All of these efforts work synergistically. I am becoming my own masterpiece one day at a time.*

## Movement:

1. I will move today.

2. I will follow my plan and make adjustments, as needed.

3. I will look for opportunities to get more use of my body while accomplishing needed daily tasks.

4. Mental health benefits of movement:

   a. Increases brain size

   b. Prevents memory loss

   c. Improves sleep

   d. Reduces anxiety and depression

   e. Boosts mood

5. Just for today, I will focus on my movement.

6. Journal thoughts, plans, or new ideas.

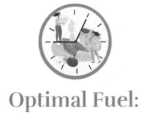

## Optimal Fuel:

1. Just for today, I will focus on the best fuel possible for the only body I will ever have.

2. I will be open to experimenting with the various foods that maximize my body's fuel. This will assure a wide variety of valuable nutrients, while keeping my meals and snacks fresh to prevent getting bored or missing important nutrients.

**3.** I will be sure to include a variety of foods daily that provide me with needed levels of fiber.

**4.** Each day I will try to learn at least one thing new about improving my body's fuel.

**5.** I will eat slowly and enjoy the food I am blessed to have.

**6.** I will put my utensil down while chewing, and I will try to avoid eating while watching television, looking at my devices, or otherwise being distracted.

**7.** I will **journal** about thoughts, plans, ideas, or concerns.

## NUTRITIONAL PEARL

**Omega 3 Healthy Benefits:**

a) Helps with depression and anxiety

b) Can help eye health

c) Can help brain health

d) Helps lower cardiac risk

e) Lowers inflammation

f) Lowers Attention-deficit/ hyperactivity disorder symptoms

**Sources of Omega 3 Fatty Acids**

a. Mackerel

b. Pecans

c. Cod liver oil

d. Flax Seeds

e. Walnuts

f. Salmon

g. Chia seeds

h. Cold pressed olive oil

i. Pumpkin seeds

j. Soybeans

k. Eggs

# Being:

## WHY LIST

1. Today, I will nurture my **Being**, just for today.

2. I am my own masterpiece, just like Pablo Picasso created his masterpiece. Each day is one brush, one dip of paint, and one stroke of the hand at a time. All the collective effort one day at a time, day after day will enhance my health and life that I can't even foresee now.

3. I will be grateful that I can move, take nourishment, and be.

**4.** I will work on my **Why List** today. I will continue to visualize each reason as I linger on each one and bask in my love or connection for them, while feeling the love or positive connection that comes back from them.

**5.** I will practice my meditative breathing today. In addition to my formal practice time, I will try to be aware of my in-breath and out-breath frequently during the day. Each time I bring this moment-to-moment awareness into my day, I am building my center of calm in the appropriate portion of my brain. These efforts will build my resilience which helps during times of suffering and pain. These unpleasant experiences come to all of us at various times. These help us withstand them more effectively and lower the probability of diverting to behaviors that lead to many of the problems we have discussed.

**6.** I will review and prepare for my unwanted behavior list. Here again, we need to develop awareness of our potential weak spots so that, if and when they arise, we can more effectively deal with them.

**7.** **Journal** thoughts, plans, and new ideas.

# DAY 11

*"Life is available only in the present moment."*

—Thich Nhat Hanh

*I will focus on **Movement, Optimal Fuel,** and **Being** today!*

# Movement:

1. I will move my body today to nourish my brain and mind.

2. Exercise promotes release of serotonin, dopamine, and norepinephrine.

3. These endorphins help to improve mood, reduce anxiety, and improve our self-esteem.

4. Daily physical activity may decrease risk of depression by 20–30 percent.

5. Daily exercise decreases the risk of dementia by 25 percent.

6. Good exercises for mental health are:

   a. Running or walking

   b. Yoga

   c. Spinning

   d. Resistance training (I will do resistance training at a level that is appropriate for my age and health status.)

7. When possible, I will do movement activities in a park or other outdoor settings as I am aware of the general additional health benefits from spending time in nature. I remain mindful of vibrant synergy for my health and well-being when I can combine activity in any two of the three categories of our program at the same time.

8. I will always consider turning on some music and dance to my tolerance and enjoyment. There are significant mind and body benefits to dancing movement while being aware of my body and what I see, hear, smell, and feel. You can do this in a group or alone if you prefer.

## Optimal Fuel:

**1.** I will give my body and mind the best nutrition possible today.

**2.** I will choose more fruits and vegetables to consume than before.

**3.** I will pick a broad array of plant colors to diversify the nutrition I put in my body today and every day!

**4.** I will consume foods rich in Omega 3 fats several times a week.

**5.** I will eat various examples of complex carbohydrates.

**6.** I will decrease consumption of red meat.

### Magnesium Benefits:

1. Decreases asthma symptoms
2. Improves memory
3. Builds healthy bones
4. Decreases muscle cramps
5. Lowers blood pressure
6. Improves heart health
7. Improves digestion
8. Decreases diabetes risk
9. Decreases anxiety and depression
10. Decreases inflammation

**NUTRITIONAL PEARL**

### Sources of Omega 3 Fatty Acids

a. Cashews
b. Sesame seeds
c. Pumpkin seeds
d. Almonds
e. Pigeon peas
f. Dark chocolate

f. Tempeh
f. Swish chard
g. Spinach
h. Soybeans

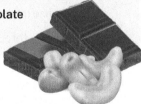

## Being:

**WHY LIST**

1. I will review my **Why I Choose to Get Healthy List**. I will linger on these reasons to help build stronger connections in the positive portion of the brain.

2. I will review my **Unwanted Behavior Trigger List.** I will visualize my relaxation and breathing response upon the unwanted appearance of a trigger.

3. I will practice my meditation breathing.

Mindfully paying attention to our senses in the present moment is an excellent way to build strength of neural synapses in the calming center of the brain. In addition, this technique can be used while walking, eating, or other activities. I do this!

I do this several times per day. I use this during mindful eating, as well as during walking and driving. I find this increases my attentiveness at that time. This slows down the rumination about past events and worrying about assumed future negative events.

## MINDFUL EATING:

1. Take a couple of slow, deep inhales and exhales.

2. Verbalize internally or externally your gratefulness for your nutrition.

3. Slowly go through your senses before, during, and after each bite.

4. It is good to lay your fork or spoon down between bites.

5. What do I see? What do I smell? What do I taste? What do I hear? What do I feel? Note any physical and/or emotional reactions.

6. Drink plenty of water or tea before the meal and between most bites.

# DAY 12

"Each morning we are born again.
What we do today is what
matters most."

—Buddha

*I will not worry about yesterday or the weeks before that. I will not think about potential obstacles or problems in the future. Today, I will focus on this day. This is my personal journey. I am unique from everyone else. I will spend each day working on my **Movement, Optimal Fuel**, and **Being**. I will be exposed to various choices in each category. My goal is to try and evaluate each one of these and choose those that feel comfortable for me. I need to make choices that speak to my body and mind and feel most comfortable for me to cultivate my **Optimal Self** on my unique journey.*

## Movement:

1. I will follow my movement plan for today.

2. I will reassess daily how my movement is helping me nourish my body and mind.

3. I will look for opportunities to vary my physical activity.

4. Where appropriate, I will do some resistance activity to tone and nourish my skeletal muscles.

5. I will look for opportunities to do good for others while doing movement that nourishes me. This could be any of a myriad of volunteer activities to raise funds for those in need, such as awareness marches, cancer fundraiser marches, mental health awareness  walks, and more. The three rewards for your participation are each very valuable:

    a. Extra physical activity

    b. Building social connections and interaction

    c. Helping others in need

All three of the previously mentioned rewards are valuable to your health and well-being, as well as to your fellow travelers along your life journey.

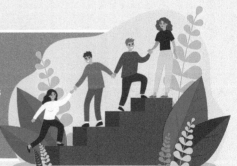

## Optimal Fuel:

**1.** Today I will focus on choosing an array of foods which will nourish my body with a broad selection of nutrients.

**2.** I will try to use different fruits and vegetables to experiment with different recipes and tastes. This will keep my meal plan fresh and interesting. I will be mindful of choosing a wide array of colored fruits and vegetables daily. This is an easy way to maximize the variation in phytonutrients consumed each day.

**3.** I will plan ahead for meals and snacks and what my plan is for each meal for the day.

**4.** I will eat less processed foods.

**5.** I am aware that if I allow myself to be without a good food choice nearby when I get hungry, I increase the probability of making bad food choices.

**6.** I will journal on my experiences today as well as new information I learn and ideas to try in the future.

**7.** I will strive to remain mindful when preparing and consuming my nutrition.

**INFORMATION PEARL**

**Magnesium:** Important in our diet due to helping regulate muscle and nerve function. It also helps with blood sugar level control and with manufacturing protein, DNA, and bones. Magnesium deficiency can cause low calcium levels as well as low potassium. Abnormal magnesium levels have been associated with diabetes, hypertension, heart disease, and osteoporosis. Symptoms of low levels of magnesium can include fatigue, muscle cramps, muscle weakness, and numbness.

## Being:

**WHY LIST**

**1.** I will practice my breathing exercises.

**2.** When possible, I will do this at free times during my day.

**3.** I know the benefits from this are additive. The more I practice, the more positive effect it has on my health and well-being.

**4.** I will review my **Why I Get Healthy List** daily.

**5.** I will be aware of my **Unwanted Behavior Trigger List.** I will practice my positive **Being** techniques to counteract negative triggers when they occur.

**6.** I will practice my breathing meditation technique during my formal set-aside contemplation/meditation time.

**7.** I will practice my **mindful eating** technique.

**8.** I know that the more I practice these techniques, the more they will help when I need to call on them when under stress or life event duress.

**9.** I will leave notes on my bathroom mirror, desk at work, or a band on my wrist to remind me to go to my **Being** techniques many times per day.

**10.** Having formal time set aside to practice is excellent. It helps to cultivate these calming centers in my brain when I do these activities more times in other settings also. The more you revisit those calming neurons and synapses, the easier it is to get into and utilize this area when you are under stress. You can build resilience to the problems of life. We all have stressful times, but the question is how you will deal with it. In all lives there are times of suffering.

**11.** **Repeated behaviors** become **habits,** and over time, I will learn to use these when stressful events or thoughts come up.

**12.** I will **journal** on my experience today and any other issues or new ideas.

# DAY 13

*"Put yourself at the top of your
to do list every single day and the
rest will fall into place."*

—Unknown

*Today I will care for myself in the best way possible. By being my best self, I am able to care for all those who I hold most dear, **one day at a time.** This is my journey, and the positive results from this day are additive to those from preceding days.*

# Movement:

1. I will follow my plan for today.

2. I'm learning how moving my body is helpful, not just for my outer physical structure, but it also has dramatic impact on my internal organs and internal biochemistry.

3. I'm learning that my brain function and mood are strongly connected to my structural body health.

4. I will look for opportunities for more Movement throughout my day.

5. I will stay open to trying other opportunities to increase my movement in ways that can also benefit my mind, body, and spirit by:

   a. Joining a group which helps me expand my community and improve my general social inter-activities and well-being.

   b. Do activities such as volunteering with organizations to help those in need.

   c. Join a dance group.

   d. Volunteer at parks or neighborhood centers.

   e. Participate in charity fundraising walks.

6. The salient point above is that increasing social interaction has vast positive impact on our general health, well-being, and longevity!

7. I will journal and evaluate where I'm at with my movement program and brainstorm adjustments or other possibilities to enhance my efforts.

## Optimal Fuel:

**1.** I will plan in advance what my meals and snacks will look like today.

**2.** I will eat, in general, what I have planned so that I will get an excellent array of nutrients.

**3.** I will have snacks available, or plan where I can get them when needed.

**4.** I will drink a good amount of water today. If possible, I will add lemon juice for its antioxidant content.

**5.** I will remember to use my Being techniques when possible while eating; this will slow down my eating process and will greatly increase my satisfaction from my meal. This will also allow me to feel full sooner with less calories consumption.

**6.** I will try to learn at least one new fact about nutrition each day.

**7.** I will journal each day my plans and any concerns or thoughts for improving the Optimal Fuel consumption portion of my program.

**8.** I will maintain my time window each day for consumption of food.

**9.** I am focusing on my nutrition just for today.

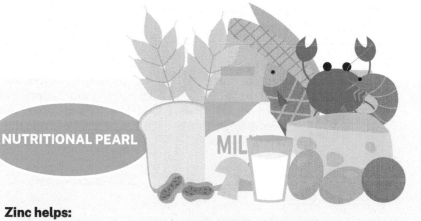

**NUTRITIONAL PEARL**

### Zinc helps:

1. Immune function
2. Gene expression
3. Wound healing
4. Protein synthesis
5. Growth and development

### Food sources of Zinc:

a. Shellfish
b. Fish
c. Nuts and seeds
d. Dairy products
e. Eggs
f. Legumes
g. Whole grains
h. Multiple vegetables

# Being:

## WHY LIST

1. Review your **Why Healthy Change List**. There is still value in writing them down, visualizing them, and lingering on them while feeling the love or connection that make each so important to you.

2. Review your **Unwanted Behavior Trigger List** and visualize your response when they happen to occur. When these triggers arise, you can deal with them by doing your mindful meditation breathing for a bit. Then, when comfortable, you can visualize the particular trigger involved by putting it in your mind's eye. You can sit with it there, and just let it be under observation. Don't try to make it go away. Just sit in awareness and let it be. You can say affirmations like, "I am safe, I am whole, emotions come and go."

3. Review your **Five Senses Meditation Breathing**. This technique can be used in many settings. You can do a walking meditation while reviewing the following questions: What do I see? What do I smell? What do I taste? What do I hear? What do I feel? You can also add: What do I feel with regard to emotion? Focusing on these senses helps you cultivate awareness of the current moment as we live it.

4. Review your **Mindful Breathing Meditation** technique. This is focusing on the breath and may include a mantra if that is your preference.

5. It is important to look for opportunities to use the above techniques not only during your set-aside meditation time, but to look for opportunities during your day to use these new skills as you are living your life. Each and every time you repeat them, you are building more connections in your brain. This will not only make you feel better more often, but it will improve your general health and increase your ability to ride the storms that come in everyone's life!

# DAY 14

"Happiness is achieved when you stop waiting for your life to begin and start making the most of the moment you are in."

—Germany Kent

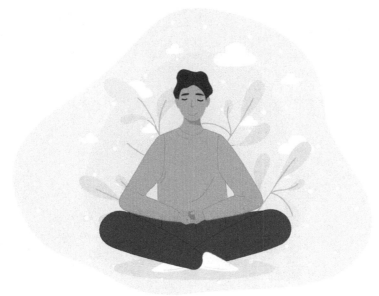

*As you begin reading this day's information, consider stopping where you are right now and take a couple slow, deep breaths. Keep your eyes open and focus on what you see. Are there colors, texture, lighting, or other things you notice?*

—

*Linger for a moment, then notice if there is anything you can smell. Is there a cologne, soap, plant, or other scent or fragrance that you can enjoy momentarily?*

—

*Next, focus on any taste you may have right now. You might have had a coffee or tea, a bagel, or breath mint or gum.*

—

*Next, focus on what you hear. There may be a radio, water running, a bird outside, or a clock ticking.*

—

*And finally, focus on what you feel. It may be your hand on your desk or lap. It may be your buttocks on your chair, your feet on the ground, or a breeze coming in the open window.*

—

*The other thing to notice is what you feel inside. It is very important to check in with this feeling regularly. Awareness allows you to use the tools you are learning to deal with your emotions in a healthier way in the long run and prevent them from being triggers for your unwanted behaviors.*

# Movement:

1. Just today, I will move my body in a healthy and enjoyable way.

2. I will look for opportunities to combine my movement with other behaviors I can do at the same time to better my health and someone else's life.

3. I might join a march or walk for a cause I believe in.

4. I may form a group or join one friend to bond with during my run, walk, or whatever activity it may be.

5. I will increase movement at times when I may have been sedentary, such as getting up from my desk and walking down the hall to the window and back.

6. I will park farther away or consider walking past my wanted item in the store before coming back to it, or I will go up and down multiple aisles in the store before checkout.

---

**INFORMATION PEARL**

### Benefits of walking include the following:

a. Longer life

b. Improves mood

c. Helps with weight loss

d. Improves sleep

e. Strengthens bones

f. Improves heart health

g. Tones and strengthens muscles

h. Lowers risk of dementia

---

# Optimal Fuel:

1. I will remember that my body and mind are the only vessels I will have through my life, and I will nourish them with the best fuel I can to function at my highest level and for the longest time possible.

2. I recognize that doing the above benefits me, those close to me that I love and cherish, and all mankind.

3. I will try to learn something new each day about fueling my body to its maximum benefit.

4. I will review the suggested foods that provide me with the greatest nutrition and please my taste buds. I will continue to look for creative ways to prepare and consume my needed nutrition.

## Being:

**WHY LIST**

1.  Each day I will exercise the techniques I am learning to help live more in the moment and spend less time ruminating about the past.

2.  At the beginning of this day's material, immediately after reading the motivational quote, I asked you to consider doing the **Five Senses Inventory**. This was noted in the general order of this workbook and that was not by accident. This was to point out that this tool is valuable to use at any time, any place, and during almost any activity. It is a way for you to keep in touch with this moment, right here, right now. The more you do this, the more you will be living in the moment, which is the only moment you have right now.

3.  Consider doing your **Why List Inventory** and, again, momentarily linger on each and relive the positive emotion it brings to you.

4.  Consider practicing your meditative breathing. This, like all the techniques, is portable and available to you at all times.

5.  Review your **Unwanted Behavior Trigger List**. Practice healthier ways to react to those negative triggers. One way to address it is during your meditative breathing. You can let the trigger linger in your awareness while continuing to focus on the breath. As you repeatedly do that over time, your trigger will tend to minimize and float away much like a bubble. This may take some time, but with repeated effort, this will be very helpful.

# DAY 15

*"Life is now. There was never a time
when your life was not now,
nor will there ever be!"*

—Eckart Tolle

*You have this day. The only thing to focus on today is,
"How will I live as the Optimal Me?" I already know this requires that
I do something today in three important areas:*

—

*I will focus on **Movement**.*

—

*I will focus on **Optimal Fuel** for my physical being.*

—

*I will focus, just for today, on **Being**, using behaviors
that will help me achieve the maximum joy, health, and sense
of well-being possible—just for today!*

# Movement:

1. Whatever movement you do, try to pick things that you enjoy doing.

2. If you are able to do some of your chores or other physical activities with friends, that is a bonus.

3. Setting aside specific time to do movement is fine. In addition, it can be helpful to extend time spent on chores or tasks of daily living. This extra movement can increase the benefits you obtain in your movement program.

4. I will stretch and warm up an appropriate amount before exercising.

5. If you have a sedentary job, you may wish to set a phone or watch alarm to remind you to get up and move around after a set period of time.

6. You could also consider setting a Fit Bit type of unit that notifies you if you don't meet a movement goal per predesignated time. An example could be 300 steps per hour. However you do it, increasing your awareness of movement and monitoring it in a way that is comfortable to you can be very helpful.

# Optimal Fuel:

**1.** I will focus on giving my mind and body the best nutrients possible today.

**2.** I am focusing just on today.

**3.** There is extensive science and evidence-based information on what benefits my physical and mental being receive when I get the best nutrition possible.

**4.** There are many examples in mainstream science of the value of studying and implementing evidence-based nutritional findings to help people improve their health and well-being.

**5.** One example of such a program is Food as Medicine: The Art and Science of Food Nutrition and Self-Healing. This is a nutritional training program by the University of California, San Diego.

**6.** Nutritional value of selected spices and herbs:

   a. Turmeric – anti-inflammatory
   b. Rosemary – anti-inflammatory, an6oxidants
   c. Parsley – rich in antioxidants
   d. Paprika – contains vitamin A and antioxidants
   e. Black Pepper – helps people to quit smoking and contains antioxidants
   f. Ginger – reduces inflammation
   g. Cinnamon – anti-inflammatory and contains antioxidants
   h. Cocoa – rich in flavonoids
   i. Garlic – contains antioxidants

**7.** Continue to **journal** on plans, thoughts, and new ideas regarding nutrition.

**8.** Each day, I will do my best to maximize the quality of the nutrition I consume.

# Being:

## WHY LIST

**1.** Today I will focus on practicing the techniques that increase my awareness of the current moment. Each time I practice, I am building the calming center of my brain which will have extensive benefits for my health and wellness.

**2.** Today, I will review my **Why Positive Change List**. I will slowly write them down, visualize each one in my mind's eye, and linger on each while feeling the positive emotional connection I have with that reason for positive change.

3. I will review my **Trigger List**, and I will visualize what techniques I will use when a particular trigger occurs. We will discuss further ways to deal with negative emotions.

4. I will review my **Breathing Exercise**. I will also remember to do this various times a day in various settings. This helps to bring it to the top of my mind so that it feels more natural to use **Relaxation Breathing** in various settings as they occur in daily life.

5. I will work on using the **Five Senses Meditation** at various times of the day. It is excellent to use while walking, particularly in nature. It is also a great way to practice mindful eating. This is an excellent exercise that is very versatile and helpful in many settings.

6. It is good to have a time set aside to practice the techniques each day, as well as use them in your daily life. The more you do it, the more benefit you will obtain.

7. The other very important point is that every time you do any of the above techniques, regardless of which one, you are training your brain to spend more time in the present. The health and well-being benefits of the change are significant and life-changing.

8. **Expressive Writing:** Expressive writing and its value with regard to enhancing health and wellness has been studied extensively by James Penneback, PhD, at the University of Texas, Austin. There are many benefits to consider for having this in your tool bag for improving your emotional and mental health. There are also many physical benefits that come from utilizing this technique. We will discuss those, tomorrow, in more detail. Today, we will give a description of how to write expressively and journal.

## EXPRESSIVE WRITING/JOURNALING

1. Pick an issue that is causing you stress, pain, or worry.

2. Write about that issue for 15–20 minutes.

3. Do this at least three to four days in a row.

4. Pay no attention to spelling, grammar, sentence structure, or punctuation.

5. Be sure to discuss emotions, including how writing this makes you feel.

6. You are writing this just for you, and need not share with anyone else.

# DAY 16

*"Make a list of what is important
to you.  Embody it."*

—Jon Kabat-Zinn

*Momentarily close your eyes and feel the breath of life enter and exit your nose. Feel the calmness. This is always available to you, any time, any place. Focus just on today. Our life journey is a series of decisions we make and actions we take, one day at a time. What we do today will be cumulative with all other days as we become our own masterpiece.*

# Movement:

1. I will follow my movement plan today.

2. I will become aware, more frequently, of how my body feels as I do various movements during my day.

3. It is good to be more aware of my muscles, joints, and structure during movement.

4. I will strive to learn more about various ways I can get in my healthy movement while also accomplishing other worthwhile tasks — things like daily chores, volunteer work, or helping a friend.

5. Don't forget to go into nature as often as you can to accomplish some of your movement plan. There are added benefits to your health and well-being as you spend time in nature. The Japanese call this forest bathing and there have been studies into the health benefits. The studies show additional decreases in stress hormone production, increased happiness, lower heart rate and blood pressure, boosting of your immune system, and accelerated recovery for injuries. So, you can increase results when doing your activity in nature. This is yet another example of the vibrant synergy of this program.

6. Consider looking into Tai Chi. It is an ancient practice from East Asia which has many benefits for body and mind health.

7. Tai Chi is an opportunity to exercise with a group of likeminded individuals and to become part of a community. This has many physical and mental health benefits.

8. Tai Chi is safe for many older individuals.

9. Tai Chi can help seniors with improving balance.

10. Tai Chi is slow and gentle and can also improve strength and flexibility.

# Optimal Fuel:

**1.** Today, I will be prepared to maximize the intake of nutritionally dense foods and to decrease the consumption of food with minimal nutrients. Many low-nutrition foods also are high in empty calories or are high in negative health substances such as trans fats or simple sugars.

**2.** I will consume a wide array of vegetables and fruits; I will look for various colors.

**3.** I will consume highly nutritious forms of protein.

**4.** I will settle and be calm to whatever degree possible each time I begin my meal until I finish. I will follow the **Five Senses Mindful Eating** when possible. This will help me to nourish and build positivity in my mind while also giving my body all the nutrients needed! This will maximize my health and well-being.

**5.** I will consume virgin olive oil daily.

**6.** I will **journal** my plans, thoughts, likes, and dislikes with my **Optimal Fuel** program.

# Being:

## WHY LIST

**1.** I will review my **Why List**.

**2.** I will review my **Unwanted Behavior Trigger List**, and I will visualize what techniques I will use to let these situations pass without negative behavior.

**3.** I will practice my breathing meditation, not only during formal practice time, but also while doing daily activities in my life. I know that this will increase the strength of my positive results over time.

**4.** The **Five Sense Mindfulness** practice is also an excellent activity I can use during various daily activities.

**5.** These activities could include:

    **a)** Walking

    **b)** Showering

    **c)** Coloring

    **d)** Doing dishes

**e)** Housework

**f)** Driving your car

*Each of the above are opportunities to bring yourself back to the here and now. Remember that life is really a series of right here, right now, moments. The more we train our mind to stay in the moment, the more enjoyment and contentment we will have with life. Importantly, this also creates many positive changes in our physiology, biochemistry, and health; it slows down aging of our DNA!*

6. **Expressive writing** health benefits per scientific evaluation include:

   **a)** Stronger immune system

   **b)** Better sleep

   **c)** Improved mental health

   **d)** Reduced pain with chronic disease

   **e)** Lower blood pressure

   **f)** Improved lung function

   **g)** Improved memory

   **h)** Improved sports performance

   **i)** Higher grade point average

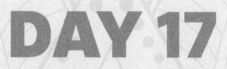

# DAY 17

*"It is never crowded along
that extra mile."*

—Wayne Dyer

*Today I will **journal** my plans, ideas, and thoughts about my*
*Movement, Optimal Fuel, and Being. Just today. Right now, this is the only*
*day I have. I will continue to incorporate the activities I'm learning into*
*my plan for today.*

—

*The more I focus on and repeat these behaviors and techniques, the more*
*positive results I will have. I will be the most optimal "me" possible.*
*Each day I will try to learn at least one new thing about*
*Movement, Optimal Fuel, and Being.*

## Movement:

1. Today I will spend time being aware and focusing on **Movement** of my physical body.

2. I will do formal exercise programs as they fit into my day.

3. I will remain aware that the additive effect of all movement is helpful.

4. I will park a little farther out, go up and down the steps more than needed, walk a bit past my destination, and turn around and come back.

5. If I'm on the phone, I will try to pace rather than sit.

6. There are safer ways for seniors to exercise but still get needed movement:

   a) Water aerobics

   b) Body weight exercises

   c) Chair yoga

   d) Walking

   e) Dumbbell weight training

   f) Resistance band workouts

   g) I would recommend seniors get some professional guidance on what is safe for their particular situation.

## Optimal Fuel:

**1.** Just today, I will be aware of trying to consume nutritionally dense foods and forego foods low in nutrients and high in simple sugars, bad fats, and empty calories.

**2.** I will consume fruits and vegetables with a broad array of colors.

**3.** I will plan ahead each day for my food plan to avoid risk of not having good choices available when hungry.

**4.** I will drink copious amounts of water as well as various teas or coffees to taste.

**5.** I will be mindful of my eating window today.

**6.** I will take two slow breaths to settle and center before eating, and I will use the **Five Senses Meditation** to be mindful and grateful for the meal I've been given.

### THE FOUR PILLARS OF THE BLUE ZONE DIET

**a)** Beans

**b)** Greens

**c)** Whole grains

**d)** Nuts and seeds

*Recall that these zones have very high percentages of their population living to over 100 years of age. They have large variations in environment and many other issues. People in these zones get a good amount of Movement and the above four foods are the common thread in diets that have some variation otherwise. I personally try to include each one of them in my diet each day.*

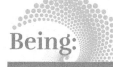

## Being:

### WHY LIST

**1.** Today, I will review and visualize my **Why List**. I will write, visualize, linger, and feel the emotional attachment to the **Why Make Positive Change** reasoning.

**2.** Today, I will be aware of my **Unwanted Negative Behavior Trigger List**. I will also be aware of the **Being** behaviors which I can use when triggers arise.

3. I will practice my **meditative breathing** today. I will also use this any time it comes to mind during my usual day.

4. I will use my **Five Senses Meditative Techniques** today. I will remain aware that this is very helpful during many activities of my day.

5. The **Five Senses Meditative Techniques** are excellent to use during my mindful eating effort. This will help me be present with each bite of my meal. I will eat more slowly. I will enjoy all the sights, smells, taste sensations, and sounds associated with my meal.

6. The more I train my mind to stay in the current moment, the more I will enjoy my life one day, one minute, one second at a time.

7. This development of awareness of moment by moment living will increase the joy and satisfaction we experience.

8. Practicing the mindful techniques for **Being** will make changes in your body which will increase your health, wellness, and probably longevity! There is evidence-based information that shows these results.

9. I will continue to **journal** and practice my **expressive writing**.

# DAY 18

*"We take care of the future by taking care of the present now."*

—Jon Kabat-Zinn

*Just today, I will focus on the only vessel I will ever have to live in. I will repeat behaviors in **Movement**, **Optimal Fuel**, and **Being**. I will practice techniques in each of these areas. I will repeat them and, over time, they will become ingrained habits that will help me become **Optimal Me**. I will focus on just today. This is my personal journey.*

## Movement:

1. Each day, my awareness of the importance of my movement to my well-being increases. During my day, I will recognize times that I could stand, walk a bit further, or take a few steps up and down stairs or inclines to improve my physical and mental well-being.

2. Resistance movement is very helpful to my health. The amount of resistance and the way it is accomplished is dependent on my level of fitness and other health-related issues. Once I am able to determine my safe zone for resistance movement, I will add that movement at appropriate times and use all necessary safety measures. A senior citizen might use a couple of cans of food to lift and move.

3. I will move today in ways that create joy and a sense of accomplishment.

4. I will consider dancing, walking, or resistance swimming.

5. I will monitor my activities in ways that allow me to be aware of progress. Examples of monitoring are counting steps, monitor time over a distance, or count reps in resistance exercise or the level of resistance itself.

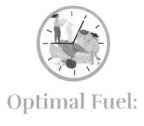

## Optimal Fuel:

1. I will plan in advance to have healthy fuel that my body needs for maximum health and well-being.

2. I will try to learn at least one new thing daily about food, nutrition, meal preparation, and how to react when a situation comes up that can lead to poor food choices.

3. I will always be aware of the triggers of unwanted

behavior, and I will know how to deal with them in a positive and productive fashion.

**4.** I will consume greens as many days as possible. In addition, I will eat a variety of fruits and vegetables. I will be mindful to make choices that assure a variety of colors in these food items each day. This will ensure that I get wide exposure to the many vitamins and other nutrients in these foods. As often as possible, I will choose fresh or frozen fruits and vegetables.

**5.** I will consume beans and legumes as many days as possible.

**6.** I will consume whole grains as many days as possible. I can eat them as a side to my meal. I can also add them to soups. I use grains such as brown rice and quinoa when I make my healthy version of fried rice.

**7.** I will consume nuts and seeds as many days as possible. Studies show that people who eat nuts and seeds tend to live longer than other people.

**HEALTHY NUTS AND SEEDS:**

a. Almonds
b. Pecans
c. Pistachios
d. Macadamia nuts
e. Walnuts

f. Brazil nuts
g. Cashews
h. Hazel nuts
i. Sesame seeds
j. Pomegranate seeds

k. Chia seeds
l. Sunflower seeds
m. Flax seeds
n. Hemp seeds
o. Pumpkin seeds

## Being:

**WHY LIST**

1. I will, each day, focus just on today. This is my personal journey.

2. I will review each of my mindful or meditative techniques daily.

3. I will use my mindful techniques each day during my usual activities whenever they come to mind and fit with that moment. This practice will increase my experience with these techniques. It will also build new neurons in the calming center of my brain. In addition, the connection between my neurons will continue to grow stronger and faster, much like

building a two-lane highway over what was once a thin dirt path between two homes.

Originally only minimal foot traffic created the path. Now the current movement and activity going through that area of my brain creates the need for the upgrade. This is what the training does in my brain over time.

4. My practice and experience in mindfulness builds an oasis of calm in my mind. It is a peaceful and private personal cocoon which is available any time and any place.

5. This center of calm is free and portable and is with me wherever I may be.

6. By repeating this behavior, physical and physiological changes will occur in my brain and mind. In addition, powerful changes will occur in my body's chemistry from practicing these techniques. This will improve a vast number of physiologic processes that will enhance my **health** and **well-being** in many ways.

7. Today I will review the **Mindfulness/Being** techniques I'm learning. I will focus more intently on the ones that speak to me and feel more comfortable for my journey. Having more skills in more areas may be helpful as various situations arise in my life.

# DAY 19

*"I am at home in my body. All is well."*

—Lois Hays

*As I awaken each morning, I will take a few slow deep breaths. I will allow my awareness to settle gently right here, right now. I will do a quick review of my focus on* **Movement, Optimal Fuel,** *and* **Being.** *Just for today.*

—

*I will set aside a few moments to* **journal** *my thoughts, plans, and feelings for this day; they are dependent on my preferences. It will be helpful to find a time of day that fits with my lifestyle and wishes. I will strive to be consistent with this. I will find, over time, this consistent and repeated journaling activity will become a habit.*

## Movement:

1. Each day, I will have a plan for my movement activity.

2. I will take the opportunity to move more than required for my work.

3. I will park further away than usual from my destination.

4. I will be sure to monitor my activity with technology, when possible, by wearing a Fit Bit or by having an app on my cell phone.

5. I will have hand weights by my chair for arm movement during television commercials or at my office desk.

   I will be aware that housework or yard work is an opportunity to increase my movement, and I will increase the frequency and level of vigor as I do these chores at a level that is appropriate for me. While doing this work I will take the opportunity to be mindful. I'll use the **Five Senses Meditative Technique** to ground my awareness in the current moment.

6. I will look for opportunities to increase community and connection with others during my movement activities. During my journaling, I will consider and write down possible community connecting activities that speak to my heart. I will further investigate the possibilities of helping others and therefore also helping myself.

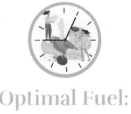

## Optimal Fuel:

1. I will plan my meals and snacks for today.

2. I will focus on foods that are high in nutritional value and that also are pleasing to my taste and general satisfaction.

3. I will try to learn one new

fact today about the benefits of one new food or item that I am considering adding to my meal plan.

**4.** I will be sure to diversify my meals in a way that prevents me from getting bored with my daily eating.

**5.** Planning is important to prevent hunger and frustration from causing us to make unwanted decisions about our fuel today.

**6.** I will be mindful and grateful for all the fuel I am blessed with.

**7.** I will focus on just today.

**HEALTH BENEFITS OF PAPRIKA:**

a) Improves blood sugars

b) Decreases inflammation

c) Decreases cholesterol

d) Improves eye health

e) Helps wounds heal

f) Helps with sleep

**HEALTH BENEFITS OF LEMON WATER:**

a) Supports heart health

b) Decreases risks of cancers

c) Decreases stress

d) Enhances immune system

e) Improves absorption of iron

# Being:

## WHY LIST

1. I will focus on just today.

2. I will review my **Why List** and linger on each reason as well as the connections I have with that reason. I will visualize each one and soak in the love and other positive emotions I receive from them or it (if not a person). I will be sure to bask in that positive energy for an adequate amount of time. Doing this will build and enhance your neurons and synaptic connections in the calming center of the brain. Over time, it will help increase the power each reason has in helping you overcome your unwanted behavior triggers.

3. I will be aware of my **Unwanted Behavior Trigger List** and will review my responses when they arise.

4. I will practice my **meditative breathing** techniques. As mentioned previously, the more you practice this behavior the more it will be easily accessible during a time of need.

5. I will be aware that I can practice this anytime and anywhere. I know that each time I do this, it solidifies my inner calm and Zen center.

6. I will practice my **Five Senses Mindfulness Technique** whenever awareness arises. This technique can be done anytime and anywhere. There are many activities that are excellent opportunities to utilize this technique:

   a) Dish washing

   b) Cleaning the house

   c) Yard work

   d) Showering

   e) Brushing teeth

   f) Puzzles and Coloring

7. It is an excellent idea to use the **Five Senses Technique** during **Movement** or **Optimal Fuel** consumption activity. When you do this over time, you are slowly moving from this being something you are doing to it becoming your way of **Being**!

# DAY 20

*"All that we are is the result of
what we have thought."*

—Buddha

*This day, right here, right now, is the only day we have. I will start the day with a few deep and slow breaths. I will focus just on today for now. I will have and follow my plan for today. I will do some **Movement**, **Optimal Fuel**, and **Being** activities.*

—

*Each day is an opportunity to learn something new. It is an opportunity to repeat, again and again, those things that, over time, will make me the **Optimal Being** I can be—right here, right now!*

# Movement:

1. I will follow my plan for today.

2. I will monitor my activities and adjust as needed.

3. I will look for opportunities to vary each activity to make it fresh.

4. I will be aware of adding my Being techniques during movement where applicable.

5. I will remember to add to my total movement for the day by being more vigorous with daily chores such as housework, yard work, and grocery shopping, among others.

6. I will also increase the time spent on these daily activities when possible.

7. Consider Tai Chi, a Chinese martial art and exercise of controlled movement.

## BENEFITS OF TAI CHI:

a) Reduces stress and depression

b) Improves mood

c) Improves energy and stamina

d) Improves balance and flexibility

e) Improves strength

f) Is safe and helpful for most seniors

g) I will remember to be mindful while doing this movement activity.

h) I will journal about my experiences, future plans, and questions with regard to this activity.

# Optimal Fuel:

**1.** Just today, I will have a plan to provide my mind, body, and spirit with the best nutrition possible.

**2.** My body and brain are the only vessels my being will ever have to live in. I will feed it accordingly.

**3.** I will include whole grains in my food plan.

**4.** Healthy fats and complex carbohydrates will be included today.

**5.** I will consume my complex carbohydrates by eating a wide variety of different fruits and vegetables of a plethora of colors.

**6.** The wider range of plants with various colors will help ensure a broad consumption of needed fiber, vitamins, minerals, and other valuable phytonutrients.

**7.** I will strive to learn one important fact about good nutrition each day.

**8.** I will remember to start each meal with a tall glass of water.

**9.** I will chew slowly and enjoy the feel, smell, taste, and appearance of my food. This Mindful approach will help me enjoy my meal more completely.

I will be able to truly savor my meal. It also will help with the digestion of all of my nutrients. Also, this will help in the general development of the calming center of the brain.

**10.** I will avoid processed foods as much as possible. Remember that most processed foods have chemicals in them that may not be nutritious. Even worse, some may be deleterious to your health.

**11.** I will do the best that I can with my food plan today. I will live life one moment and one day at a time.

**12.** I will journal about my nutrition today.

# Being:

## WHY LIST

1. I will review my **Why List**. I will write, visualize and linger over each item on the list. I will savor the positive emotion of each one to help counteract negative behavior triggers when they may arise.

2. I will review my **Unwanted Behavior Trigger List**. I want to remain aware of those issues which may encourage me to fall off my program. You may

choose to use the **Self-Compassion Awareness Meditation** (see at the end of this chapter).

3. I will review my **meditative breathing** exercises.

4. I will review my **Five Senses Mindful/Meditation** practice.

5. I will, each day, strive to recognize times during my usual daily activities when I can use at least one of the above **Being** techniques. The more I practice, the better the results I will get.

6. I will remember that each practice session will lead to more and larger brain cells in the calming center of the brain. These increasingly larger neurons will also increase in size and connection to each other. I will remember the analogy of the bicep of one arm growing larger after curling a dumbbell time after time, day after day.

7. Over time, with practice of these helpful techniques, they will become a true part of our **Being**.

## SELF-COMPASSION AWARENESS MEDITATION

1. Notice or become aware of negative emotion.

2. Relax and take some deep slow breaths.

3. Shift your awareness to how you feel.

4. You may put your hand on your heart, which helps release oxytocin, the hormone of safety.

5. Empathize with your experience.

    a) "This is hard."

    b) "This is upsetting."

    c) "This is painful"

    d) "This is scary."

6. Give yourself compassion.

    a) "May I be kind to myself."

    b) "May I accept this as it is."

    c) "May I give myself compassion."

    d) "May I accept myself as I am."

7. Continue the above until you feel a shift from the negative emotion.

# DAY 21

*"Learn to appreciate what you have
and where and who you are."*

—Wayne Dyer

*I will be grateful that I have been given another day. I will continue to learn something new each day. I will focus on becoming the **Optimal Me!** Each day, I will strive to combine **Movement, Optimal Fuel,** and **Being** techniques in ways that are pleasing. I will remember that there is a vibrant synergy between three areas that enhance and complete **health** and **well-being.***

# Movement:

1.  I will have a plan for movement for today.

2.  I am aware that there is value in the accumulation of movement across my day.

3.  I will find multiple opportunities during the course of my day to increase my movement when accomplishing a task or chore.

4.  I will remember that movement does more than nurture my bones, muscles, ligaments, tendons, and joints.

5.  Movement will lower my risk of many chronic diseases, including Alzheimer's, heart disease, diabetes, cancer, anxiety, and depression.

6.  Remember that daily chores can be part of your movement plan. You can increase speed or distance of movement for additional benefit. You can take more steps, repeat lifting, and repeat bending or stretching.

---
**BENEFITS OF SWIMMING:**

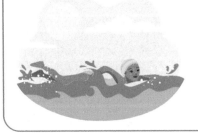

1.  Helps with stress, anxiety, and depression
2.  Helps burn significant calories
3.  Helps lower the risk of chronic disease like heart disease or diabetes
4.  Helps with energy levels and sleep

## Optimal Fuel:

**1.** I will plan my day's consumption of the best fuel possible for my body and mind.

**2.** I will strive to learn something new each day about selecting foods that are nutrient-dense and calorically low.

**3.** I will strive to consume my fuel as mindfully as possible. I understand that part of the vibrant synergy for this lifestyle is that time and choices in each of our three areas, when combined, will lead to healthy **behaviors** that will become **habits.** They are engrained in us at this point.

**4.** **The Five Senses Meditative Technique** is excellent to use while eating my meal.

**5.** By diversifying my food each day, I will make sure that I am getting an excellent array of required nutrients.

**6.** Items that are always in my refrigerator include: greens, carrots, celery, multicolor peppers, mushrooms, hummus, coffee, green tea, red wine vinegar, apple cider vinegar, onions, feta cheese crumbs, a Rotisserie chicken, skim milk, low salt soy sauce, Kefir, low fat plain 100 percent Greek yogurt, and milled flax seeds.

**7.** I will continually review the **Do and Do Not Recommendations** from Day 2 of this program. I want my repeated choices from this program to become my habits.

**8.** I will remember that it can be helpful to consume some low-calorie nourishment at the beginning of my meal, which will help decrease my appetite to a degree, as well as help me manage one of my personal issues. This is particularly helpful if you are a compulsive eater. It is most helpful early in my journey to becoming **Optimal Me.**

## Being:

### WHY LIST

**1.** I will continue to touch base and review the previous suggested behaviors and techniques.

**2.** I will review my **Why List**.

**3.** I will review my **Unwanted Behavior Trigger List**.

**4.** I will practice my **Focused Breathing Meditation.**

**5.** I will practice my **Five Senses Mindful/Meditative Technique.**

**6.** I will stay aware to combine **Movement** activity or **Optimal Fuel** activities with my **Being** techniques. This is when the **vibrant synergy** of these techniques and behaviors become even more powerful. They become much more than what you are doing, they become what you are!

**7.** Remember the analogy of Pablo Picasso using various simple techniques again and again to create **YOUR** masterpiece. This happens one day at a time.

**8.** I am focusing on one day at a time.

**9.** Consider keeping a **Gratefulness Journal**; here are the benefits:

   **a)** It causes positivity.

   **b)** It improves self-esteem.

   **c)** It reduces stress.

   **d)** It makes you happier.

   **e)** It helps you sleep better.

   **f)** It shifts your focus from the negative to the positive in your life.

   **g)** It improves your quality of life.

   **h)** It reduces your inner most fears.

   **i)** It enhances your faith.

   **j)** It helps you reach your goals.

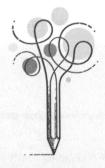

**INFORMATION PEARL**

**HOW DO YOU WRITE IN THE JOURNAL?**

**a)** Short sentences

**b)** Bullet points

**c)** Use more detail over time.

**d)** Write each idea as it pops in your head.

Remember that this is a 30-day workbook that is presenting a lot of valuable information. It is not probable that you will be able to or want to do everything mentioned each and every day.

The goal is to always remember this is **YOUR journey**. No two are alike. You need to consider and try as many suggestions in this book as possible, then focus more on the ones that really speak to your inner self.

You should do as comprehensive a program as possible each day within the three main areas, Movement, **Optimal Fuel, and Being**. You should try to do as much as possible from each area that connects with you in a visceral way and has the **vibrant synergy** for your **health** and **well-being**.

# DAY 22

*"The goal is not to be better than the other man, but your previous self."*

—Dalai Lama

*I will be grateful for all that I have been blessed with this day. I will journal my plans, thoughts, and possible areas of further study. I will remain aware that this book will expose me to different concepts and techniques. It is up to me to practice them and determine which techniques feel comfortable to me. I will practice those that speak to my heart and physical **Being**. This is my journey. I need to strive each day to do something in each group—**Movement, Optimal Fuel,** and **Being!** The power is in doing something in each one daily.*

## Movement:

1. I will begin my day with a plan for movement.

2. I will be aware of my fitness level and will do what is safe for me. I will cautiously increase my activity level.

3. I will look for opportunities to diversify movement to keep it fresh. I will participate in a community movement program when possible.

4. While I'm moving, I will remember to bring mindful awareness to the activity. There is a tremendous opportunity to bring mindful awareness to movement activity. This is how the vibrant synergy of this program will develop and help change your life.

5. If you are more senior or have particular disabilities that limit your movement, don't overlook a movement program in a pool. Many facilities have such classes, and it's a great way to get a safe and stable movement activity in a relaxing environment.

6. There are many benefits to daily walking:

    a) Improves probability of a longer life

    b) Helps to bolster brain function

    c) Contributes to weight loss

    d) Can help lower risk of vision problems like cataracts

    e) Improves mood

    f) Lowers risk of hypertension and diabetes

    g) Strengthens muscles and bones

## Optimal Fuel:

**1.** I will have a plan for the day, and I will follow my plan.

**2.** I will have access to healthy snacks to help avoid making poor nutritional choices at times of stress or unforeseen hunger.

**3.** I will strive to consume a wide variety of nutrients with various fruits and vegetables of different colors and nutritional content.

**4.** I will focus on my nutritional plan just for today.

**5.** I will try to learn something new each day about optimal nutrition.

**6.** I will plan to have snacks available that are nutritious and fit into my Optimal Fuel program.

**7.** I will drink an appropriate amount of water daily.

I will also drink tea or coffee seasoned to taste. I will avoid all fruit juices and other artificial beverages because most have large amounts of simple sugars and other non-healthy additives.

**8.** I will remember to season my foods with many of the spices we have discussed. They will not only increase my foods flavoring, but they are also very nutritionally dense which can augment the health value of my meals.

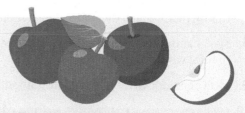

**HEALTH BENEFITS OF APPLES:**

**1.** High in water and fiber

**2.** Contain manganese, copper, vitamins A, E, B, B2

**3.** Help with weight loss

**4.** Have polyphenols for antioxidant effects

**5.** Help to lower risk of diabetes

**6.** Have probiotics for gut health

**7.** May lower risk of cancer

## Being:

**WHY LIST**

**1.** I will today focus on the various **Being** techniques I am learning and practicing.

**2.** These techniques help me to be more aware of my day, right here and right now.

3. These efforts produce positive effects which are dose dependent. The more I practice these techniques, the more positive effect they will have on my total health and well-being.

4. I will review my **Why List**.

5. I will review my **Unwanted Behavior Trigger List**. I will review my approach to dealing with them.

6. Today, I will do my breathing meditation, not only during formal set-aside time, but at any time it comes to top-of-mind awareness. This, like my other techniques, will provide benefits in direct proportion to the amount of time they are used. I will try to bring awareness to my everyday activities as I work, play, and do other general activities.

7. I will review my **Five Senses Mindful/Meditation Techniques**. I will remain aware that using this technique trains my brain and mind to spend more time on awareness of the here and now. This technique is something I can do during much of my daily life when it comes to mind.

8. I will meld these activities into my daily life so they become more of my natural way of **Being**.

9. I will consider writing in my **journal** today.

10. I will practice my **expressive writing** while working in my journal. I will recall the health and well-being benefits of this type of writing.

11. I will practice my **Gratefulness List**.

12. Today is the only day that I am focusing on. This is my personal journey. I know that the more often I can have my awareness on the current moment instead of thinking about previous events or possible negative events in the future, my health will benefit in multitudes of ways.

# DAY 23

*"Every morning we are born again.
What we do today is what
matters most."*

—Buddha

*Today is the only day I really have. I cannot change yesterday or the day before that. I will focus on **Movement**, **Optimal Fuel**, and **Being**. I will become my best self, one day at a time. Each positive behavior has the same effect on my well-being as each curl of the dumbbell has on the bicep of the weight lifter.*

# Movement:

1. I will focus on movement today. It will be nourishing for my body, mind, brain, and emotional being.

2. Whatever movement I participate in, I will bring my awareness to what I am doing. I will notice the nourishment going to my muscles, joints, bones, heart, and brain.

3. I will stay aware that as I focus on the sensations of nourishment going to my physical being, I am also building stronger connections in the calming portion of the brain. This is the synergy of **Movement, Optimal Fuel**, and **Being** each day!

4. I will try to schedule walking meetings. If this is doable in nature, that is even better.

5. I will try to do stretching a few times per day.

6. I will take the stairs more often.

7. I will do more household chores more often and for longer periods of time.

8. I will dance more often. I will turn on music that speaks to me and then move my body while bringing awareness to the activity as I do it.

9. I will monitor and track my steps or miles per day as well as repetitions of things like stretching. Keeping track of performance is a good way to see how I'm progressing.

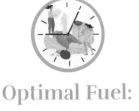

# Optimal Fuel:

1. Just today, I will focus on maximizing the quality of the fuel that I consume.

2. I will be mindful of the pleasure

I receive from this nourishment in addition to what it does in my body.

3. I will linger on the sight, smell,

taste, feel, and sound of the nutrients as I consume them.

**4.** I will journal about my experiences, and I will develop and follow my plan for today.

**5.** Today I will learn at least one new thing about nutrition and food, as well its preparation.

**6.** I will focus on today!

**7.** I will have a plan for today and have healthy food and snacks available to decrease the possibility of making poor Optimal Fuel choices.

**WHAT IS KEFIR?**

**1.** A fermented drink made from kefir grain and milk

**2.** Contains a combination of live bacteria and yeast to cause fermentation.

**3.** Evidence-based benefits:
   a. Good for digestion
   b. Rich in calcium
   c. More protein than an egg
   d. Supports your immune system

## Being:

### WHY LIST

**1.** I will focus on today.

**2.** I will remember that at any time of the day, I can add to my health and well-being by being aware of that current moment. I will consider having cues placed at locations like my desk at work, in my car, on my shower door, or any location where I often spend time that will bring my attention to my breath and allow me to be mindful in these normal daily activities. Ultimately, this repetitive behavior will engrain **Mindful Living** into being my habit.

**3.** I will check in with my breath or mantra as a way to be aware of the current moment. This will slow down the continual fixation on the looping video of previous events in my life.

**4.** This current awareness will also slow down the constant worry over perceived possible negative events in the future.

**5.** I will continue to review the various techniques I am learning. The more I practice them and use them in real situations, the more engrained they will become in my mind. There is a physical change that occurs in the brain, as well as growing resilience to life's challenges and ups and downs.

**6.** I will review my **Why Make Healthy Change List**.

**7.** I will review my **Unwanted Behavior Trigger List**.

**8.** I will review my **Mindfulness Meditation Technique**.

**9.** I will review my **Five Senses Mindful/Meditation Technique**.

**10.** I will review my **expressive writing**.

**11.** I will review my **Gratefulness List** journaling.

# DAY 24

*"Let us try to recognize the precious
nature of each day."*

—Dalai Lama

*I will be grateful that I awoke again today. Today I will do **Movement**, consume **Optimal Fuel**, and again practice **Being**.*

—

*I will begin today right where I am. I am my own masterpiece. Each positive behavior is one more paint stroke on the canvas of my best life. I am my masterpiece.*

## Movement:

1.  I will have a plan for movement today.

2.  I will mix up my movement to keep it fresh.

3.  I will do movement that not only speaks to my body structure, but also provides relaxation and joy.

4.  I will remain aware of increasing activity of daily work or chores.

5.  I will do movement outside and in nature. I will be aware of the benefits of exposure to nature on a regular basis. If I do movement in nature and add mindful activity to the session, I will again create a vibrant synergy of health and wellness benefits.

6.  I will remain aware that when I do this again and again, I am, over time, going from doing well-being activities to being well-being. This repetition will become a habit, our **Being**, and our way of life.

7.  If my health status will support it, I will try to get a couple episodes of vigorous movement for 10 or 15 minutes about 2 or 3 times weekly. A faster pace walking or a slight incline might accomplish this goal.

8.  I will try to do some stretching often prior to movement. I will strive to be mindful with all these activities.

9.  I will do some resistance movement 2 or 3 times per week.

## Optimal Fuel:

1. I will focus just on today.

2. I will have a plan for today that I will follow to the best of my ability.

3. Preparation is key.

4. I will consider having snacks available at all times to prevent me from getting cravings to consume foods that are not on my plan.

5. Depending on my daily schedule, I will carry snacks with me, if possible.

**6.** I will consume a good amount of various multicolored fruits and vegetables daily. This will assure me of a large amount of the vitamins and other nutrients that are critical to have my body and mind functioning at its Optimal level.

**7.** I may want to consider taking a cooler in my vehicle to carry nutritious snacks or meals such as lunch.

**8.** I will also look for a food store if I am short of foods to snack on or eat for a meal.

**9.** Some foods available for a quick meal from the grocery store include:

a) Yogurt

b) Kefir

c) Packaged fish like salmon, tuna, sardines

d) Raw vegetables including:

  i.   Carrots

  ii.  Celery

  iii. Tomatoes

  iv. Spinach

  v.  Hummus

  vi. Various fruits

  vii. Nut butter or nuts and seeds

  viii. Packaged beans

**10.** You may want to keep some paper plates/bowls/silverware on hand as well as a can opener for meal stops at grocery stores.

**11.** You can often find some healthy options at the deli section of the store. Many have various healthy salad options as well as lean meats or grilled fish.

**12.** I will be mindful during my meal, and I will avoid multitasking. I will use the appropriate techniques that I have been learning to accomplish this.

## Being:

**WHY LIST**

1. I will remember each of the tools I have been exposed to, and I will continue to use them during formal practice time. I will also practice them where appropriate during other daily activities.

2. I will be aware that using these techniques during my daily activities will continue to help build resilience to the ups and downs of life.

These different activities have positive effects on my health and well-being in a dose-dependent way. The more I practice, the more significant positive impacts these exercises will have on me. This is the vibrant synergy of focusing on behavior from each of the three areas we are stressing each day — **one day at a time!**

3.  The activities from the **Being** section will help me build more connections in the calming portion of the brain with more powerful connections built between them. This is known as neuroplasticity, and it significantly improves my total health.

4.  I will journal my experiences with **Movement** and **Optimal Fuel** today.

    I will review and practice each technique I've learned to the best degree possible.

# DAY 25

*"Without exception, begin every day with gratitude."*

—Wayne Dyer

*I will begin today with gratitude. I will center myself on having a laser focus on just today. I will nurture my awareness on the three areas of* **Movement, Optimal Fuel,** *and* **Being.** *I will have a plan. I will do whatever preparation is needed for a successful day. No matter how long the journey, it is still one step after another.*

—

As a young boy, I used to dream of walking the Appalachian Trail. The trail is 2,190 miles long, start to finish. It takes the average hiker 5 to 7 months to complete the whole trail. Only about 25 percent of those attempting to complete the whole trail actually achieve it. This, in many ways, is analogous to our life journey. We have some idea of where we would like to end up. The reality is we don't know for sure if we will achieve that goal. There are three things we control that we know we can do. The first is to plan and prepare ourselves to the best of our ability so that we have the best opportunity possible to achieve our goal. The second part is to help ourselves develop the ability to savor every moment of whatever time and distance we DO have on the trail. The final part is to develop ourselves so that what we leave behind all along our path will be better than it was before we got there.

## Movement:

1. I will have plans for movement today.

2. I will stand and stretch more often.

3. I will stand and walk while talking on my telephone.

4. I will take the stairs.

5. I will park further away.

6. If I leave my desk at work, I will walk a little further after my chore before returning to my desk.

7. I will consider taking a walk through nature today.

8. When sitting and watching television, I will have something of weight nearby to move with my arms.

**9.** I will contact a friend to take a walk and have a conversation.

**10.** In good weather, I will spend more time in my yard or at someone's home who needs help doing chores and thereby getting more physical activity.

**11.** I will be sure to accomplish whatever movement activity I have planned for today.

**12.** I will remember to bring my awareness to the moment of my physical activity, and I will use that opportunity to be aware and be present during that physical activity.

# Optimal Fuel:

**1.** I will have a plan for this day's nutrition. Life is one day at a time!

**2.** I will be sure to have high nutritional value foods and snacks available today. I will also strive to avoid highly processed foods, foods high in simple sugars, or any foods containing trans fats.

**3.** I will spend some time while shopping in the store making note of foods that would make good choices if I'm traveling and need a quick meal or snack.

**4.** I will remember to avoid soft drinks and fruit juices since they usually contain simple sugars and often other unhealthy chemicals.

**5.** I will eat less manufactured and processed foods.

**6.** I will get a broad array of plants to eat daily. This will broaden the nutrients consumed and keep my body and mind at their peak health and well-being.

**7.** I will try to consume fruits and vegetables as near to their raw state as possible.

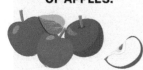

**BENEFITS OF APPLES:**

**1.** High in fiber

**2.** High in vitamin C

**3.** Low in calories

**4.** High in polyphenols, which is an antioxidant

**5.** Can lower risk of Alzheimer's, cardiovascular disease, and Type 2 Diabetes

**6.** Lowers risk of many gastrointestinal diseases

# Being:

## WHY LIST

1. I will review the techniques I have learned from previous chapters, and I will repeat them often.

2. I will remember that each time I practice a technique, I am building actual physical changes in my brain and body.

3. These changes will help me build a better sense of well-being and calm on a daily basis. They also will help me build resilience in times of stress, confusion, or pain. All lives have these periods of emotional pain or challenges.

4. I will focus on meditative and mindful practices just for today.

5. I will consider doing mindful eating.

6. I will consider doing mindful walking.

7. I will consider being mindful during my shower.

8. I will consider being mindful when doing chores such as washing dishes or vacuuming.

9. I will remember that mindfulness meditation is helpful for other issues, such as enhancing the microbiome, which plays a key part in many other health and wellness issues.

10. Just this day, I will realize that each time I practice mindfulness, it is just like the weightlifter doing arm curls with a barbell. The results are dose dependent.

# DAY 26

*"Meditation makes the entire nervous system go into a field of coherence."*

—Deepak Chopra

*I will focus, today, on integrating these new behaviors into my daily tasks. As I do this one day at a time, my well-being will improve just like a lake is formed, by each rain drop that falls time after time. I will look for opportunities to do well for others as I am doing well for myself.*

## Movement:

1. I will focus on increasing my movement today.

2. I will look for ways to increase my movement that's enjoyable to me.

3. I will look for opportunities to help others while also nurturing my own well-being with **Movement**.

4. I may decide to pick up a side gig near my home where I can increase physical activity while also helping someone in need. This could be as a volunteer or through extra income. An example would be helping a senior citizen with yard work, dog walking, or other chores as needed.

5. I will look for groups doing activities that appeal to me and allow me to improve my well-being by building community.

6. With inclement weather, I may go to a shopping mall or large store to walk on a safe, dry surface and have easy access to clean and safe restroom facilities. When the weather is inclement enough, I go from one store to another just to get in a walk in a safe and dry setting.

7. I will be aware of stairs with a handrail to possibly use for an increased intensity work out that is safe for me if I have any stability concerns. Again, I should not do any physical activity that my health-care provider does not feel is safe for me. I will be sure to get cleared first.

**BENEFITS OF PICKLEBALL:**

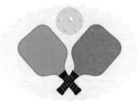

1. Boosts mental health and mood
2. Helps burn calories
3. Results in fewer injuries/is low impact
4. Improves balance and agility
5. Good for bones and muscles
6. Helps build social/community connections

# Optimal Fuel:

**1.** I will have a plan for maximizing the quality of the nutrition I consume today.

**2.** I will focus on today only.

**3.** I will continue to learn something new each day about what foods are both pleasing and satisfying to me.

**4.** I will have access to snacks and quality food if something happens in my day to increase stress or unwanted behaviors.

**5.** I will express my gratitude for my nourishment.

**6.** I will take a couple slow and deep breaths to center myself.

**7.** I will put down my utensil while chewing and savoring my meal.

**8.** I will use this opportunity to be mindful while eating. I will appreciate the vibrant synergy this creates for my health and well-being at mealtime:

   a. I will express gratitude.
   b. I will take a couple slow deep breaths and I will focus:

   - What do I see?
   - What do I smell?
   - What do I taste?
   - What do I hear?
   - What do I feel?

   c. I will remember the feel can be tactile and/or emotion!

**9.** I will consider trying a food which is known to be nutritionally optimal but is something I have not tried before.

**10.** I will keep in mind to switch out animal-based protein with plant-based protein. There are health benefits that occur the more often we consume plant-based nutrition.

# Being:

## WHY LIST

**1.** I will focus just on today!

**2.** I will **journal** if this touches me at my core.

**3.** I will review my **Why Positive Change List**.

**4.** I will review my **Unwanted Behavior Trigger List**.

**5.** I will consider doing my breath exercises/meditation.

**6.** I will consider doing my **Five Senses Mindful Meditative Practice**.

**7.** I will consider keeping my **Gratefulness Journal**.

**8.** I will integrate the above techniques in my daily living to the degree that they speak to me.

**9.** **Loving Kindness Meditation:** A type of meditation that cultivates kindness for all beings, including your family and yourself, decreases illness, and increases well-being. The benefits are:

a) Increases compassion

b) Increases empathy

c) Decreases bias toward others

d) Increases social connections

e) Reduces self-criticism

f) Helpful even in small doses

g) Has long-term positive impacts on the practitioner

h) Helps you be more helpful for people

i) Slows biological aging (by increasing telomeres length)

j) Increases parasympathetic control-relaxation

k) Increases gray matter in emotion part of the brain

l) Helps brain's emotional processing

m) Decreases schizophrenic spectrum disorder

n) Decreases PTSD

o) Decreases chronic pain

p) Decreases migraines

q) Increases positive emotions and decreases negative emotions

**10.** Now that I have some background information on **Loving Kindness Meditation**, I will practice this tomorrow.

**11.** To repeat this book's ongoing premise, this is **YOUR** journey! You are layering tools to you for your practice, consideration, and determination of how each fits with you!

**12.** There is no expectation or requirement that you use each technique every single day. You are being exposed to multiple brushes, paint colors, types of paint strokes, and canvas types. You will develop skills as additional tools in your toolbox as needed. You will choose the tools to make your unique masterpiece. We will go through the **Loving Kindness Meditation** tomorrow, Day 27.

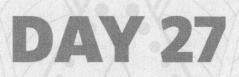

# DAY 27

*"Be kind wherever possible,
it is always possible."*

—Dalai Lama

*I will be kind to myself today. I will journal, learn, and practice (just for today) self-care.  By doing **Movement**, **Optimal Fuel**, and **Being**, I am being kind to myself. This will provide me the opportunity to be kind to others. That kindness will spread like the ripple from a stone thrown into a pond. You never know what difference that kindness will make in another's life today.*

# Movement:

1. Today, I will have a movement plan, and I will follow it.

2. I will be mindful of my level of fitness and will use caution about increasing my movement intensity too quickly.

3. I will be aware of the value of using the techniques I'm learning from the **Being** section during my movement.

4. I will remember that repetition, over time, will help to change random **behaviors** into **habits.**

5. I will constantly look for ways to increase my physical activity when completing activity at work, home chores, or relaxation time.

6. My efforts' rewards are additive. I am focused just on this day, right here, right now.

7. I may shoot baskets, mow the neighbor's lawn, or participate in walks that raise awareness or funds for causes that I believe in and support.

8. I will be mindful to stretch, bend, and reach often. I will pay attention to what I see, hear, and feel while I do this. This will help me to be grounded in this moment.

9. If I am a golfer, I will consider walking during my round.

10. I will consider riding my bicycle.

## Optimal Fuel:

1. I will focus on my nutritional intake just for today.

2. I will have a plan, and I will follow it.

3. I will try to learn one new fact about nutrition today.

4. I will strive to choose a wide variety of foods in

each of the **Do Choose** categories in our **Optimal Fuel Plan**.

**5.** A wide array of colors are best when choosing vegetables and fruits to broaden the nutrient intake.

**6.** I will remain aware of the value of using the **Five Senses Mindful Meditation**

during **Optimal Fuel** consumption. Each effort in this regard is addictive in the positive effects on my physical, biochemical, and neurological health and well-being.

**7.** Best foods for brain health:

a) Fatty fish
b) Coffee
c) Blueberries
d) Turmeric
e) Broccoli
f) Pumpkin seeds
g) Dark chocolate
h) Nuts
i) Oranges
j) Eggs
k) Green tea

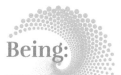

# Being:

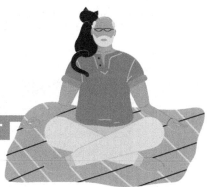

## WHY LIST

1. I will focus just on today!

2. I will journal my thoughts and plans.

3. I will review my **Why Get Healthy** list.

4. I will review my **Unwanted Behavior Trigger List**.

5. I will practice my **Mindful Breathing Meditation**. I will also use this at various times during my day as I become aware of it, and if it seems appropriate with whatever I am doing.

6. I will review my **Five Senses Meditation**, and I will use this as feels appropriate. This could be during driving, walking, eating, showering, washing dishes, or other chores.

7. I will complete my **Gratefulness Journal**.

8. I will learn more about the **Loving Kindness Meditation**.

## MEDITATION

This is a powerful meditation that helps us build compassion, empathy, and goodwill toward ourselves and others we know and may not know. Yesterday's **Being** section discussed many of its positive effects. Today, we will go through the details of this simple but powerful meditation.

**FIRST, WE START WITH A SERIES OF POSITIVE AFFIRMATIONS:**

**1.** May you be safe. May you be protected.

**2.** May you be free of internal and external harm.

**3.** May you be happy and content.

**4.** May you be healthy and whole to whatever degree possible.

**5.** May you experience ease of well-being.

**Loving Kindness Meditation** is very powerful. Research shows regular use of this meditation creates many positive effects for the practitioner.

You can use it just referring to yourself as a way to increase self-compassion. You also can start with you saying, "May I ...." and say the affirmations. You can then visualize people you love and send the positive energy to them. That can be followed by someone neutral, then someone you've had strained relations with. Finally, you can send it to all mankind. The repeating of this meditation over time will reward you in many ways.

# DAY 28

*"Self-discipline is self-caring."*

—M. Scott Peck, MD

*As I repeat the behaviors I learn one day at a time, I will slowly make powerful changes in myself. Physiological, biochemical, and structural changes will occur. My structures will get stronger. I will be adding more brain cells in the calming center of the brain, and the connections between brain cells will become stronger. My immune system will improve. Just like raindrops added to a lake, my self-discipline and self-caring will have positive effects on my health and well-Being.*

# Movement:

1. I will focus only on this day!

2. I have a plan for today. I will follow the plan.

3. I will monitor length and intensity of my activity.

4. I will diversify my activity when possible, to broaden my physical and emotional pleasure.

5. When possible, I will take opportunities to do activities while also building community connections. The stronger connections I develop with others, the more my health and well-being will improve.

6. If my health and fitness level allows it, I will do a bit more intensive aerobic activity for 10–30 minutes, 2–3 times per week, which will add additional benefits to my health. If it is warranted, I will get an evaluation and recommendation from my health provider on the appropriate level and intensity of exercise for me.

7. Some type of weight lifting or other resistance exercise two days per week is also helpful.

8. Aerobic exercise has been shown to be particularly helpful in preventing dementia. Any exercise can be helpful to some degree in that regard.

9. I will practice **Being** techniques during **Movement** when possible.

10. I will always be aware that any opportunity to do my movement in nature has other added well-being benefits.

11. I will do my **journaling**.

## Optimal Fuel:

**1.** I will have a plan for getting my healthy meals and snacks today.

**2.** I will focus on just this day.

**3.** I will be sure to vary the color of my fruits and vegetables to help in getting the array of nutrients I need to maintain optimal health.

**4.** I will cut back on the amount of red meat I eat, if I eat it at all. I will be sure to consume only the leanest cuts of meat and limit my portion sizes.

**5.** I will strive to eat more plant-based food.

**6.** I will consume less prepackaged and manufactured foods and attempt to increase the amount of fresh or frozen plants that I eat. I will eat more fruits and vegetables that require minimal preparation prior to consumption by me. This will increase the number of phytonutrients that I consume. These phytonutrients are very healthy for my body and mind.

**7.** I will be mindful with food preparation and with meal consumption.

**8.** When I sit to eat, I will:

a. Take a couple deep breaths
b. Be grateful for my meal and give thanks
c. Be aware of the experience and how it makes me feel:

- What do I see?
- What do I smell?
- What do I taste?
- What do I hear?
- What do I feel? Tactile feelings? Hunger? Stress? Safety?

## Being:

**WHY LIST**

**1.** I will focus just on today, minute by minute, right here, right now.

**2.** I will continue to bring my attention or awareness to this moment, one moment at a time.

**3.** I will review the previous techniques from this book, and I will visualize myself going through them.

**4.** I will visualize myself using these techniques as I go through my various activities of daily living.

*The more I use these techniques during other activities, such as taking a shower, washing dishes, walking, running, or any number of others, I will be combining mindfulness with that activity. You will find, over time, you will immediately attach mindfulness to the active movement. This helps you live in the moment! You will spend less time on the never-ending movie loop of previous life events in your mind and constant worry about possible negative events in the future. When this happens, you will have more resilience against the inevitable problems of life.*

5. I will consider reviewing my **Why List** and make any needed adjustments.

6. I will consider reviewing my **Unwanted Behavior Trigger** List.

7. I will consider reviewing and practice my **Breath Meditation**.

8. I will consider reviewing and practicing my **Five Senses Mindful Meditation** technique.

9. I will consider reviewing my expressive writing.

10. I will consider reviewing my gratefulness journaling.

11. I will consider reviewing my **Loving Kindness Meditation**.

12. I will do my **journaling**.

# DAY 29

*"Pain is certain, suffering is optional."*

—Buddha

*I will focus today on learning, practicing, doing, and repeating the behaviors of this book that speak to me. I am aware there will be obstacles. There will be times of pain. It is part of the human condition. I know that I am learning and changing in ways that will help me ride out the hurricanes of life and continue to thrive to the best of my ability. I will* **journal** *my experiences, thoughts, and plans.*

## Movement:

1. I have a plan for movement today.

2. I am following my plan for movement.

3. I will stretch often.

4. While moving, I will drop into awareness of my senses.

5. I will consider using a rubber ball to grasp repeatedly. I know that repeated grasping will help build hand strength.

6. I will consider standing, walking, and stretching on commercial breaks while watching television or working on my computer or digital device.

7. When I go to the mailbox or any other errand, I will consider going a bit further and come back to my actual destination.

8. I am aware that movement is addictive in its positive effect on my health, wellness, and general well-being!

9. Movement is not only helpful for my external body, but it is also very beneficial for my internal organs like my heart, lungs, and even brain!

10. Increasing movement will also lower my risk of chronic diseases such as Alzheimer's, cancers, diabetes, and cardiovascular disease.

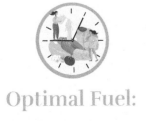

## Optimal Fuel:

1. I will focus on just today in getting the maximal amount of nutrients in my body.

2. I will focus on consuming quality sources of protein.

3. I will strive to increase my consumption of plant-based foods. They are an excellent source of protein as well as complex

carbohydrates, fiber, and other vitamins and phytonutrients.

**4.** I will focus on drinking enough water to stay well hydrated. I will also consume coffee and tea to taste and tolerance.

**5.** I will continue to approach my eating from a mindful perspective.

**6.** I will express my gratitude for my nutrition.

**7.** I will start with a couple of deep breaths.

**8.** I will diversify my diet plan to the degree needed to keep my meal time

exciting and enjoyable. I will try to learn at least one new piece of information daily on healthy foods. I will always strive to improve the Optimal Fuel I consume.

**9.** I will express my gratitude for my food as well as my life.

**10.** I will take one bite at a time. I will put down my utensil and chew more than in the past.

**11.** I will choose from a wide array of fruits and vegetables.

**12.** I will frequently use as a common base of meals:

a) Beans of all varieties
b) Greens
c) Whole grains
d) Nuts and seeds

**13.** I will consume fermented foods frequently to maintain a robust microbiome. This is very important for my immune system, brain health, and many other important physiological functions.

**14.** I will go through my Five Senses Mindful techniques while eating to improve my health and decrease the likelihood of emotional eating.

## Being:

**WHY LIST**

1. **Loving Kindness Meditation**

    a) The longer version of this would be to first refer to yourself with the pronoun "I."

    b) Next you can move on to referring to someone you have a strong attachment to using the "may you be" term. You can go through as many of these as you like.

    c) Then you can pick someone you are neutral toward and wish them well with the same phrasing.

    d) Next you can choose someone you are not close with or have had diffculties with. You can repeat this with as many people as you like.

**e)** Finally for an ending, you can refer to a global group like the country, world, or universe.

*This meditation very quickly helps to improve many well-being markers as we've previously discussed.*

**2.** I will review my **Why Healthy Change List**.

**3.** I will review my **Trigger of Unwanted Behavior List**.

**4.** I will review my **Five Senses Mindful Meditation Technique**.

**5.** I will review my **Breathing Meditation Technique**.

**6.** I will review my **expressive writing exercise**.

**7.** I will review my **Gratefulness List**.

**8.** I am aware that today is but one day on my personal journey. This is my journey and it is unique to me. My best use of this book is to continue to review and practice the material that speaks to my heart and mind. As I develop my personal preferences under each of the three categories and repeat them over and over, I will become the product of those positive behaviors.

# DAY 30

*"Give yourself permission to allow
this moment to be exactly as it is and
allow yourself to be exactly as you are."*

—Jon Kabat-Zinn

*Like every day before, this current day is all that we have, right here and right now. I accept today just as I am. I will continue to work on becoming more resilient to life's storms and challenges. I will continue to focus on one day at a time!*

# Movement:

1. I have a plan for **Movement** today.

2. I will use caution in increasing the level of intensity or time in my movement program to decrease the risk of harm.

3. I will continue to experiment with different types of movement. I know this will keep my interest and enjoyment fresh. I will also be diversifying the positive effects of my movement by doing different types of movement.

4. I will continue to practice my awareness during my movement. I can monitor this by using the **Five Senses Technique:** What do I see, smell, taste, hear, and feel? I could also just focus in on one area, such as paying attention to the movement of my body, what I'm seeing, or what I'm hearing. I can focus on just being aware.

5. I will consider combining community interaction with some movement.

6. I will focus only on the movement plan that I will participate in today. I will choose something that speaks to me and nourishes my mind and spirit as well as my physical being.

7. I will stretch and warm up appropriately prior to my activity.

8. I will include resistance, general movement (like walking or whatever is appropriate), and two to three episodes of more intense activity during your week. Clearly, there is a wide variation from person to person as to which movement is appropriate and to what level of intensity. Don't be hesitant to discuss with your physician or another professional about what is appropriate for you.

# Optimal Fuel:

**1.** I have a plan that will assure I consume a wide variety of nutrients that will provide my mind and body with a broad array of nutrients.

**2.** I will strive to cultivate a mindful attitude while consuming my nutrition today. Optimal Fuel this day is just for today!

**3.** I will be aware of eating a majority of my nutrition from plant-based sources.

**4.** I will strive to learn one new fact today about good nutrition.

**5.** I will be prepared for snacks and choices I can easily make if my schedule changes or I become hungry at an unusual time.

**6.** I will try to use fruits and vegetables in inventive ways to diversify my plant-based consumption. I will obtain as wide an array of plant-based foods as possible.

**7.** I will not make my choices of plant-based foods based only on the taste. I will also focus on nutritional value, diversification of the various phytonutrients, and general impact on optimizing my health and wellness.

**8.** I will avoid food that contains simple sugars. I will also avoid white bread, regular potatoes, and white rice. These are reduced quickly to simple sugar when consumed.

# Being:

## WHY LIST

Below is a list of the Being techniques that we have reviewed over these 30 days. The last one we present today. Acts of kindness are self-explanatory. There are many benefits to making this part of your day. It is a very easy thing to do and has large benefits.

**1.** Why Make Healthy Changes Inventory

**2.** Triggers of Unwanted Behaviors Inventory

**3.** Mindful Breathing Meditation

**4.** Five Senses Mindful Meditation

**5.** Daily Journaling

**6.** Gratefulness List

**7.** Expressive Writing

**8.** Loving Kindness Meditation

**9.** Acts of Kindness

*Acts of kindness have many benefits:*

**a)** Releases oxytocin, the love hormone which helps the heart

**b)** Increases energy

**c)** Increases happiness

**d)** Increases lifespan

**e)** Increases pleasure

**f)** Increases serotonin, an antidepressant brain chemical

**g)** Decreases physical pain

**h)** Decreases stress

**i)** Decreases anxiety

**j)** Decreases depression

**k)** Decreases blood pressure

**l)** Even witnessing acts of kindness have some benefit.

---

*I will circle back to the way we started this 30-day workbook. Over this 30-day period, we have focused on living one day at a time. Each day, we strive to have a plan in three areas, **Movement**, **Optimal Fuel**, and **Being**. We have evaluated much information in each area. The beginning goal of this process was to learn and practice different techniques in each of the three areas. Ultimately we pick the ones that speak to our heart and soul and feel right for our own life journey. As we continue to live our program day by day, moment by moment, we begin to not just be **doing** these behaviors, but we also **become** them. As these habits develop and grow in us, this truly becomes our **Being**. In addition, these physical and biochemical changes have a **vibrant synergy** which has profound effects on our health and well-being. There is a great increase in the probability of adding years to our life, and life to our years. In addition, these changes in ourselves will help us have a positive* *effect on many around us. I like to use the visual of throwing pebbles in the water and watching the ripples move out. We can create much positivity, some of which we may not even be aware of. We may not know other positive effects it is causing further down the line.*

*That's what this book means to me. I am more grateful and feel more blessed than I can even express. From where I was, to where I am today, is an amazing journey. I want to use my journey to benefit others. I will spend the rest of my time helping as many people as I can to become the most **Optimal Person** that they want to be and can become. Who knows how far the ripples from my pebbles thrown in the water will travel? Please share this work with anyone who might benefit.*

*Gratefully,*
*Dwight*

# EPILOGUE

This book contains a lot of important and powerful information. The more you follow these suggestions, the more positive effect you will have.

✿

You could focus on each day's information for more time before proceeding.

✿

You may decide to spend 2 days on each day's material before you proceed, or you could work straight through then do it again.

✿

You will notice much repetition, and this is by design. The more you work on something the more engrained it becomes.

✿

Repeated behaviors become habits, and repeated habits can become traits.

✿

I encourage you to journal, each day, your thoughts, plans, or issues that come up in each of your three focus areas: Movement, Optimal Fuel, and Being.

✿

Preparation and planning are key to success.

✿

Your journey is your journey.

✿

Live one day at a time!

becomingoptimalyou.com

Made in the USA
Columbia, SC
14 May 2022

60303401R00085